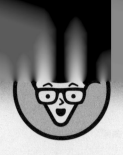

Quick Diabetic
Recipes

D1202487

by American Diabetes Association®

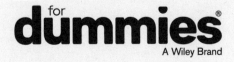

for
dummies®
A Wiley Brand

Quick Diabetic Recipes For Dummies®

Published by: **John Wiley & Sons, Inc.**, 111 River Street, Hoboken, NJ 07030-5774, www.wiley.com

Copyright © 2018 by John Wiley & Sons, Inc., Hoboken, New Jersey

Published simultaneously in Canada

For general information on our other products and services, please contact our Customer Care Department within the U.S. at 877-762-2974, outside the U.S. at 317-572-3993, or fax 317-572-4002. For technical support, please visit https://hub.wiley.com/community/support/dummies.

Wiley publishes in a variety of print and electronic formats and by print-on-demand. Some material included with standard print versions of this book may not be included in e-books or in print-on-demand. If this book refers to media such as a CD or DVD that is not included in the version you purchased, you may download this material at http://booksupport.wiley.com. For more information about Wiley products, visit www.wiley.com.

Library of Congress Control Number: 2017961508

ISBN 978-1-119-36323-1 (pbk); ISBN 978-1-119-36327-9 (ebk); ISBN 978-1-119-36328-6 (ebk)

Manufactured in the United States of America

10 9 8 7 6 5 4 3 2 1

Contents at a Glance

Recipes at a Glance

Table of Contents

Introduction

A diabetes diagnosis can be surprising and incredibly intimidating. If you or a loved one has just been diagnosed with diabetes, you may be feeling overwhelmed. You're not alone! Many Americans are affected by diabetes, either directly or through friends and/or family members who have this chronic disease. In fact, according to the Centers for Disease Control and Prevention, an estimated 23.1 million Americans were living with a diagnosis of diabetes in 2015. The good news is that diabetes can be managed. There is a lot you can do to keep yourself healthy, including building a healthcare team, balancing the food you eat with exercise and diabetes medications (if prescribed), and taking care of your mental well-being.

When you have diabetes, you're responsible for your own care. But you may be wondering where to begin. First things first: Learn everything you can about diabetes and the different aspects of diabetes care. Find reliable information about diabetes online or in self-care guides, ask questions at your next doctor's appointment, or request a referral to a diabetes education program. Knowledge is power, so make sure you're prepared with all the information you need.

You'll also need to make some changes to what and how much you eat. This can be a big adjustment for most people, but good nutrition is essential to successful diabetes management. Understanding what, how much, and when to eat with diabetes can be challenging in the beginning, especially if you're not familiar with diabetes nutrition. Fortunately, resources and experts — doctors, dietitians, and diabetes educators — are available to help you. By selecting this guide to diabetes cooking and meal planning, you've already taken your first step toward eating and living well with diabetes.

About This Book

Think of your diabetes diagnosis as an opportunity to live a healthier lifestyle. This book is the perfect guide to help you begin making healthier food choices and cooking delicious diabetes-friendly recipes at home. This book may have the word *recipes* in the title, but it's so much more than your average cookbook. You find out about the best food choices for diabetes, the basics of diabetes nutrition, how to find a meal plan that works for you, and how to shop for and prepare healthier recipes.

This book primarily covers type 2 diabetes, but people with type 1 diabetes and gestational diabetes can also benefit from the tips and techniques in the pages ahead and enjoy these easy-to-prepare recipes. We hope this guide will become a trusted resource for you to turn to when you have questions about diabetes nutrition or are looking for a satisfying meal for any occasion.

Each easy-to-follow recipe in this book features a serving size and prep and cooking times so you know exactly what to expect before you begin cooking. Complete nutrition information is provided for each recipe as well, so you know exactly how a dish will fit into your meal plan. You'll also find some tips in the recipe chapters that will make the cooking process even easier; some recipes include possible variations so you can put your own spin on them.

As you make the recipes, keep the following points in mind:

>> All herbs are fresh unless dried herbs are specified.

>> All temperatures are Fahrenheit.

>> Read through a recipe completely before you begin cooking to make sure you have all of the ingredients and equipment you need.

🍅 The tomato icon highlights vegetarian recipes in the Recipes in This Chapter section on the opening page of each chapter, as well as in the Recipes at a Glance.

The nutrition and meal planning information in this book is not intended to serve as a replacement for meeting with a dietitian or diabetes educator. Instead, think of it as a primer to prepare you for your appointment with a professional and a reference to help you make healthy food choices. Use this guide to discover the variety of meal-planning approaches that can work for people with diabetes and then meet with a dietitian or another diabetes care provider to discuss which option will work best for you.

Foolish Assumptions

If you're reading this book, you probably have diabetes or are close to someone who does. Maybe you have just been diagnosed and need to figure out what to eat with diabetes. You may not have had a chance to meet with a dietitian or diabetes educator yet. Or perhaps you're caring for a spouse, parent, or child who has diabetes and you want to get a better understanding of this disease and how to cook for them. You don't need to be familiar with diabetes nutrition to benefit from this book. We cover the basics for you!

Maybe you already have an understanding of what to eat with diabetes but you're interested in learning how to cook diabetes-friendly meals at home, or you're looking for new dishes to spice up your meal plan. The recipes in this book are great for beginner and experienced cooks alike. And if you think you don't have time to prepare healthy meals from scratch, think again. Some recipes take longer to prepare than others, but the recipes in this book were created for the busy person with diabetes. We understand that spending hours in the kitchen isn't practical for everyone, but cooking at home can be a much healthier (and tastier) alternative to ordering takeout or relying on prepackaged meals. Whatever your schedule or skill level in the kitchen may be, you'll find recipes in this book that are perfect for you!

Icons Used in This Book

You'll find icons throughout this book that alert you to helpful information, facts to remember, and technical information that may help if you're looking for a more advanced understanding of the topic.

TIP

The Tip icon marks important information that can save you time and energy as you're planning, shopping for, and preparing diabetes-friendly meals.

REMEMBER

When you see the Remember icon, it means the information is essential and you should be aware of it.

WARNING

The Warning icon warns about potential problems that you may want to consider. It's often used to alert you to how certain foods may impact your body or meal plan.

TECHNICAL STUFF

The Technical Stuff icon gives you technical information that may be helpful, but is not necessary, to your understanding of the topic at hand. You can skip over this information, if you want.

Beyond the Book

In addition to the book you're reading right now, be sure to check out the free online Cheat Sheet for details on the best food choices for people with diabetes, tips for smart grocery shopping, and a list of ways to prepare before you start cooking. To get this Cheat Sheet, simply go to www.dummies.com and type **Quick Diabetic Recipes For Dummies Cheat Sheet** in the Search box.

Where to Go from Here

It's time to get started planning and preparing incredible, healthy meals! Take a moment to read through the Table of Contents and explore all the topics that this book has to offer. Where you start is up to you. If managing diabetes is new for you, Chapter 1 provides a great overview of the best food choices for people with diabetes. Interested in the meal planning, carbohydrate counting, or portion control techniques? Turn to the chapters in Part 5 for an introduction to these topics. Looking for tips on shopping for healthy foods or stocking your pantry? Chapters 2 and 3 have you covered. The information in Parts 1, 4, and 5 can give you the knowledge you need to choose tasty and nutritious foods, understand how to manage your diabetes with your diet, and feel confident in the kitchen. If you're using this book as a guide to meal planning with diabetes, remember to consult with a dietitian or another diabetes care expert to determine which meal-planning approach is right for you.

If you already have a good grasp on what to eat with diabetes, have a meal plan in place, or have some experience cooking at home, then grab an apron and dive right in to the recipe chapters! Find a recipe that sounds appealing to you and start cooking. If you're looking for a hearty breakfast option, for example, check out the recipes in Chapter 4. Want to impress your friends with a fun and healthy appetizer for your next get-together? Jump ahead to Chapter 10. There's a recipe in this book to fit every mood, palate, and occasion!

You don't need to read this book from cover to cover or visit the chapters in any particular order to benefit from the information in this book. Instead, use it as a reference to get more information about the topics that are important to you and find recipes that suit your tastes and get you excited about eating well with diabetes.

Whether you're just learning about diabetes or you've been successfully managing your diabetes for years, this book is your go-to reference for all your food-related diabetes questions. This collection of straightforward and delicious recipes is sure to become a favorite in your home. We hope you'll return to it again and again throughout your journey with diabetes and that it brings some comfort and joy to your kitchen.

1
Getting Started with Diabetic Cooking

Chapter **1**

What Can I Eat?

O ne of the most common questions that people with diabetes ask is, "What can I eat?" Being aware of what you eat when you have diabetes is important for keeping blood glucose levels in your target ranges and reducing the risk of complications. This task can be overwhelming, especially for people who have just been diagnosed. But living with diabetes doesn't mean you have to feel deprived, overhaul your whole diet, or stop eating the foods you love. It's about choosing nutritious foods and preparing them in a way that is healthy and enjoyable. When you know the basics of healthy eating, it gets easier! You'll be cooking flavorful, satisfying, nutrient-rich meals in no time.

The great news for people with diabetes is that a huge variety of healthy and delicious food options are available. Having diabetes can be an opportunity to embrace healthy eating.

In this chapter, we explore six food categories — vegetables, fruits, whole grains, protein, fat, and dairy — and identify the best food options within these categories for people with diabetes.

Introducing the Importance of Carbohydrates

Knowing what to eat when you have diabetes can be very confusing, especially in today's world where fad diets, food trends, and "miracle" foods are advertised everywhere you look. You're bombarded with ever changing and often conflicting information about what you "should" and "shouldn't" eat. Don't let all this information overwhelm you! Many nutrition basics for people with diabetes have withstood the test of time.

Before we take a look at some of the foods that will set you up for diabetes management success, we need to give you a brief introduction to a nutrient that is very important for people with diabetes: carbohydrate. Three main nutrients (or macronutrients) — carbohydrate, protein, and fat — make up all the foods we eat. *Carbohydrate* is a nutrient found in fruits, vegetables, grains, milk and yogurt, and starchy and sugary foods and drinks. Carbohydrate is the nutrient that raises blood glucose levels, so it's important for people with diabetes to be aware of their carbohydrate intake. But carbohydrate should not be completely removed from your diet; your body needs a certain amount of carbohydrate to function properly.

As you work your way through this chapter, you'll see that many of the best food choices for people with diabetes contain carbohydrates. Carbohydrates are not the enemy! The important thing is to choose nutrient-rich sources of carbohydrate rather than refined, sugary carbohydrates. For more information on carbohydrate and other macronutrients, see Chapter 16.

Eat Your Vegetables!

You may remember your parents making sure you ate all the vegetables on your plate when you were young. That's because vegetables are full of vitamins, minerals, fiber, and other nutrients, and they're often relatively low in calories and carbohydrate (the primary nutrient in foods that affect blood glucose — see Chapter 16 for more information); this makes them great for people with diabetes — and everyone else!

But not all vegetables are created equal. Vegetables can be divided into two main groups: nonstarchy and starchy. Starchy vegetables contain more starch and, therefore, more calories and carbohydrate than nonstarchy vegetables. Both kinds of vegetables are an important part of a well-balanced diet, but starchy vegetables have an impact on blood glucose. So, if you have diabetes, moderation is important when it comes to starchy vegetables.

Nonstarchy vegetables

Nonstarchy vegetables are a great way to satisfy your appetite. Enjoy these vegetables often! When it comes to nonstarchy vegetables, more is better (which is not something you hear very often when you have diabetes). Try to eat three to five servings of nonstarchy vegetables per day; this will help you get the vitamins, minerals, and fiber you need to stay healthy. Some common nonstarchy vegetables include the following:

Artichokes and artichoke hearts	Leeks
Asparagus	Mushrooms
Beets	Okra
Bok choy	Onions
Brussels sprouts	Pea pods
Broccoli	Peppers
Cabbage (all varieties)	Radishes
Carrots	Salad greens (arugula, endive, escarole, lettuce, radicchio, romaine, spinach, watercress)
Cauliflower	
Celery	Sprouts
Cucumber	
Eggplant	Squash (crookneck, spaghetti, summer, zucchini)
Greens (all varieties)	Tomatoes
Green beans	

TIP

You can enjoy fresh, frozen, or canned varieties of any nonstarchy vegetable. When it comes to canned or frozen vegetables, the best choices for people with diabetes are varieties without added sodium, sugar, or fat. Purchase canned vegetables that say "low sodium" or "no salt added" on the label. If you have to use canned vegetables with sodium, drain and rinse them before cooking to reduce the amount of sodium. Try to limit or avoid frozen or canned vegetables that come in sauces; they tend to be higher in fat and sodium.

Starchy vegetables

When you have diabetes and want to eat starchy foods, try to choose the most nutritious starches available instead of eating processed, refined starches. Starchy vegetables are a great option. They contain fiber and nutrients that are good for your body. They'll raise your blood glucose due to their carbohydrate content, so moderation is important.

The best starchy vegetable choices for people with diabetes are those without any added salt, sugar, or fat. Common examples of starchy vegetables include the following:

Acorn squash	Parsnips
Butternut squash	Potatoes and sweet potatoes
Corn	Pumpkin
Green peas	

An Apple a Day . . .

Fruits are another healthy food choice for people with diabetes. Fruits contain carbohydrate and affect your blood glucose, so be sure to account for them in your meal plan (see Part 4). But they're also full of fiber and nutrients that a health body needs. If you have a sweet tooth, great news: A serving of fruit is a wonderful alternative to heavier desserts and sugary treats.

The best fruit choices for people with diabetes are fresh, canned, and frozen fruits without added sugars. When shopping for canned fruits, look for options that are packed in juice or light syrup. Here are just a few examples of the many fruits you can enjoy:

Apples	Melon (cantaloupe, honeydew, watermelon)
Apricots	Oranges
Avocados	Papaya
Bananas	Peaches
Blackberries	Pears
Blueberries	Pineapple
Cherries	Plums
Grapefruit	Raspberries
Grapes	Strawberries
Kiwi	
Mangoes	

TIP

Dried fruits such as cranberries, dates, figs, and raisins are another option for people with diabetes. They make a handy and tasty snack. But dried fruits are usually high in sugar, so the serving sizes are small. Dried fruits are just concentrated versions of fresh fruits — think about the size of a raisin compared to a grape, or a prune compared to a plum. So watch your portions if you choose to add dried fruits to your diet.

Making Your Grains Count

Wondering if people with diabetes can eat starchy foods like grains and pasta? Yes, they can! The key to including starches into your diet is to make them count. This means choosing the most nutritious starches available instead of filling up on processed starches with little to no nutritional value. So, ditch the refined grains, sugary starches, and white-flour-based products! The better bet is to choose whole grains and whole-grain products.

A *whole grain* is an entire, unrefined grain. Whole grains are made up of the bran, germ, and endosperm of the grain, which contain a lot of nutrients. Refined grains have been processed to remove parts of the grain, and are missing many of the nutrients of their whole-grain counterparts. So, for a fiber and nutrient boost, try replacing the processed grain products on your plate with whole grains or whole-grain products. Switch out that white rice for brown or wild rice. Look for breads and pastas that are made with 100 percent whole-wheat flour. Or experiment with whole grains like quinoa, barley, or farro.

Some popular whole grains to try include the following:

Brown rice	Quinoa
Bulgur or cracked wheat	Sorghum
Buckwheat or buckwheat flour	Whole farro
Corn meal and whole corn	Whole-grain barley
Millet	Whole rye
Oatmeal and whole oats	Whole-wheat flour
Popcorn	Wild rice

TIP

When shopping for whole-grain foods, make sure you check the food labels. You'll see many products in your grocery store that claim to be made with or contain whole grains. But don't let clever packaging fool you; some products that make these claims actually contain only a small amount of whole grains. Check the ingredient list and choose foods that have a whole grain or whole-grain flour listed as the first ingredient.

TIP

The Oldways Whole Grain Council has created a Whole Grain Stamp to make it easier for consumers to spot products that contain at least half a serving of whole grains. This stamp features a sheaf of grain on a golden-yellow background, and there are three varieties of the stamp that indicate different amounts of whole grain. For more information on the Whole Grain Stamp, visit www.wholegrainscouncil.org/ whole-grain-stamp.

Choosing Lean Protein

Protein foods are another important part of a well-balanced, diabetes-friendly diet. A wide variety of protein options — from poultry to seafood to plant-based proteins like tofu, beans, and lentils — are great for people with diabetes.

The important things to consider when choosing protein foods are the fat content of animal-based proteins and the carbohydrate content of plant-based proteins. When it comes to protein, keep it lean; people with diabetes should avoid too much fat in their diets because eating too much fat, especially saturated fat and trans fat, can lead to weight gain and increase the risk of heart disease. The best protein choices for people with diabetes are poultry, fish, and other seafood that is not fried, as well as plant-based proteins. Eggs, egg whites, and egg substitutes are other good options.

Poultry

Poultry is a relatively lean source of animal-based protein, but it still contains saturated fat and cholesterol. To cut down on some of the excess fat, choose skinless cuts of poultry when shopping or remove the skin before cooking and try to choose white meat cuts (breasts and tenderloins) instead of the slightly fattier dark meat. Chicken, turkey, and Cornish game hens are all good poultry options. Duck contains more fat than chicken and turkey, so if you enjoy duck, keep that in mind.

Fish and seafood

Seafood is another type of lean protein that is great for people with diabetes. Fish containing omega-3 fatty acids (a beneficial type of fat) are especially good options. Types of fish that are high in omega-3 fatty acids include albacore tuna, herring, mackerel, rainbow trout, salmon, and sardines. (For more information on omega-3 fatty acids, see Chapter 16.) Other fish and seafood options to enjoy include the following:

Catfish	Halibut
Clams	Lobster
Cod	Oysters
Crab	Scallops
Flounder	Shrimp
Haddock	Tilapia

WARNING

Keep in mind that some fish are high in mercury and should be enjoyed in moderation or in some cases avoided all together. This is especially important for pregnant and breastfeeding women and small children. If you're concerned about the mercury content of a certain fish, you can check the Food and Drug Administration and Environmental Protection Agency's consumer advisory about fish. Visit www.fda.gov/downloads/Food/FoodborneIllnessContaminants/Metals/UCM537120.pdf. Fish choices that have the highest mercury content and should be avoided include the following:

Bigeye tuna (sometimes labeled as "ahi")	Orange roughy
	Shark
King mackerel	Swordfish
Marlin	Tilefish

Plant-based proteins

If you're not very familiar with plant-based proteins, it's time to explore this wonderful protein option. In addition to providing protein, the foods in this category also provide fiber (which you don't get from animal-based proteins), and many contain healthy fats. These added nutritional benefits are a great reason to incorporate plant sources of protein into your diet. However, just like fruits, vegetables, and grains, plant-based proteins do contain carbohydrate and will affect your blood glucose; make sure you read nutrition labels for these products and account for the carbohydrate in your diabetes meal plan (see Part 4).

So, what are plant-based proteins? This type of protein includes beans, lentils, peas, soy, and nuts, as well as products made from these foods. Here are a few delicious plant-based proteins you can try:

Beans (black, kidney, pinto, and so on)

Bean products (baked beans, bean burgers, refried beans)

Chickpeas

Edamame

Hummus

Lentils (all varieties)

Meat replacement products (meatless chicken, bacon, beef, burgers, hotdogs, and so on)

Nuts and nut spreads and butters

Peas (black-eyed peas, split peas)

Soy nuts

Tempeh and tofu

TIP

Meat substitutes, such as meatless burgers, soy "chicken," and other foods, have become more popular in recent years, especially with vegetarians. You'll see a wide variety of meat substitutes available in your local grocery store, and many of these meatless proteins are tasty and easy to prepare. Feel free to try these products, but keep in mind that they may be higher in carbohydrate than their meat counterparts and may contain sodium and unhealthy saturated fats. It's a good idea to check the nutrition labels on these products before making a purchase.

Plant-based proteins are an excellent choice for people with diabetes, so dig in! Just remember that unlike other forms of protein, plant-based proteins contain carbohydrate and will affect your blood glucose. Checking food labels will help you learn the serving sizes of plant-based proteins and understand how they fit into your diet.

Red meats

What about red meat? Are beef, pork, and lamb okay to eat for people with diabetes? The short answer is yes. But red meats and pork are generally higher in saturated fat than other forms of protein. So, enjoy these meats in moderation and try to choose the leanest options available. Look for high-quality grades of meat and try to purchase cuts that have been trimmed of fat. Some of the better choices when it comes to red meats include the following:

>> **Beef:** Chuck steaks, cubed beef, flank steaks, porterhouse steaks, rib, round, rump roast, sirloin, and T-bone steaks

>> **Game:** Bison, rabbit, venison

>> **Lamb:** Chop, leg, or roast

>> **Veal:** Loin chops or roast

- **>> Pork:** Center loin chop, ham, tenderloin
- **>> Organ meats:** Hearts, kidneys, and livers

You have lots of options when it comes to red meats. And you'll find several healthy and delicious beef, pork, and lamb recipes in Chapter 8. But it's important to be mindful of the fat content of these meats when you have diabetes. Choosing leaner proteins like chicken, seafood, or plant-based proteins for most of your meals can help reduce your risk of high cholesterol and heart disease.

Fat: Good or Bad?

Are fats healthy or unhealthy for people with diabetes? You may have heard a lot of conflicting information about fat. Fat has a bad reputation for being harmful, but believe it or not, your body needs fat to function properly, and there are healthy fats. We're here to help explain the difference between various types of fat. By the end of this section, you'll have a better understanding of how fats fit into a healthy lifestyle with diabetes.

Fat may be the second most important nutrient for people with diabetes to monitor in their diets behind carbohydrate. The fat you eat has an effect on weight management, which is a goal for many people with type 2 diabetes, and cardiovascular health. All fats, regardless of type, are high in calories, so it's important to keep an eye on portion size when eating foods that contain fat.

REMEMBER

The *type* of fat you eat is more important that the total amount of fat. There are healthy and unhealthy kinds of fat. Healthy fats include unsaturated fats (both monounsaturated and polyunsaturated) and omega-3 fatty acids; these fats have heart-protective properties. Cardiovascular (heart and blood vessel) complications are a concern for people with diabetes; limiting the intake of saturated and trans fats — the unhealthy fats — and choosing healthy fats instead is a step toward reducing the risk of heart disease in people with diabetes.

The following sections give you some examples of each kind of fat to help you understand which fat-containing foods to incorporate into your diet and which foods you may want to avoid.

Unhealthy fats

Saturated and trans fats are known as the unhealthy fats. Saturated fats raise your blood cholesterol levels, which is a risk factor for heart disease. People with diabetes are already at an increased risk for cardiovascular complications, but you can help protect your heart by eating less saturated fat and replacing the sources of saturated and trans fats in your diet with healthy fats. But the first step toward making that change is to identify the sources of unhealthy fats. Some examples of foods that contain saturated fats include the following:

» Butter

» Cream and cream sauces

» Chocolate

» Coconut and coconut oil

» Fatback

» Full-fat dairy products (cheese, ice cream, sour cream, whole and 2 percent milk)

» Gravies

» High-fat, highly processed meat (bacon, ground beef, hotdogs, sausage, spareribs)

» Lard

» Palm oil and palm kernel oil

» Poultry skin

Limiting these foods can reduce your risk of heart disease. A general goal is to aim for less than 10 percent of your daily calories to come from saturated fat, which amounts to roughly 13–22 grams of saturated fat per day depending on your calorie needs. Check with your healthcare provider or a registered dietitian (RD) or registered dietitian nutritionist (RDN) to see if this goal is appropriate for you. When shopping for fat-containing foods, check the nutrition label; foods with 1 gram of saturated fat or less are generally considered low in saturated fat.

Trans fats, also called trans fatty acids, are processed fats that are created by turning liquid fats, such as vegetable oils, into solid fats. There are naturally occurring trans fats, but most trans fats you see in products on the market are added to foods during processing. The primary source of trans fats is partially hydrogenated oil. Trans fats used to be found in many products, including margarines and butterlike spreads and baked goods such as biscuits, cakes, cookies, frozen pizza, and pie crusts. Trans fats are being removed from the food supply because, in 2015, the U.S. Food and Drug Administration determined that trans fats were not "generally recognized as safe." Food manufacturers have until 2018 to fully remove trans fats from foods. Generally speaking, all people should avoid trans fats. So, check food labels and look for products with zero trans fats.

Healthy fats

Monounsaturated fats, polyunsaturated fats, and omega-3 fatty acids are healthier choices than saturated and trans fats (see the preceding section). Monounsaturated and polyunsaturated fats are considered healthy because they have the ability to lower LDL or bad cholesterol. This is great news for people with diabetes (and the general population) because high LDL cholesterol is a risk factor for cardiovascular complications. Sources of unsaturated fats include vegetables, nuts, and seeds.

You'll find monounsaturated fats in the following foods:

>> Avocados

>> Canola oil

>> Nuts (almonds, cashews, peanuts, and so on)

>> Olives and olive oil

>> Peanut butter and peanut oil

>> Sesame seeds

Sources of polyunsaturated fats include the following:

>> Corn oil

>> Cottonseed oil

>> Mayonnaise

>> Pumpkin seeds

>> Safflower oil

>> Salad dressings

>> Soft margarines

>> Soybean oil

>> Sunflower oil and seeds

>> Walnuts

Omega-3 fatty acids can improve heart health by reducing the risk of clogged arteries. The primary sources of omega-3 fatty acids are fish and some plant foods — canola oil, flaxseeds and flaxseed oil, soybean products, and walnuts. Fish that are high in omega-3 fatty acids include the following:

>> Albacore tuna

>> Herring

>> Mackerel

>> Rainbow trout

>> Salmon

>> Sardines

So, enjoy a few servings of (nonfried) fish per week to take advantage of the benefits of heart-healthy omega-3 fatty acids!

The Do's and Don'ts of Dairy

Dairy products contain calcium and vitamins that are important for a healthy body. Including dairy in your diet is a great way to build strong bones and get some high-quality protein. But dairy products also contain saturated fat (see the "Unhealthy fats" section earlier in this chapter), so it's important to pay attention to the serving sizes of these products. Low-fat and fat-free milks and yogurts may be good dairy choices for people with diabetes, especially when chosen instead of higher-fat options like half and half, cream, butter, cheese, and sour cream. If you don't like milk or are lactose intolerant, fortified milk substitutes such as almond milk, soymilk, or rice milk can be a good source of calcium and vitamin D.

TIP

If you're used to higher-fat dairy products, it may take a little while to get used to the taste of low-fat dairy. You can make the transition slowly. For example, if you use whole milk in your coffee or cereal in the morning, try switching to 2 percent milk and then transition to fat-free milk if you choose.

What Can I Drink?

Just as some foods are better for you than others when you have diabetes, some drinks are better for you than others. The drinks you choose can either support or hinder your healthy food choices.

REMEMBER

Don't forget the nutrients in your drinks! Liquid calories and carbohydrates still count and can affect your blood glucose and weight. Choose the best drink options to keep your healthy eating on track.

Steering clear of sugary beverages

Drinks that are sweetened with sugar such as regular sodas, fruit drinks and juices, energy drinks, and sweet teas will increase your blood glucose faster than most foods and can make it much harder to get to your blood glucose goals. If you love regular sodas, you're not alone; reducing soda intake is a goal for many people who are diagnosed with type 2 diabetes. But it's important to choose zero- or very low-calorie drinks instead of regular sodas. Each serving of regular soda contains a large amount of carbohydrates, which raises your blood glucose, and can contribute more than 100 calories to your diet. These numbers add up! Just a few servings of high-calorie, high-carbohydrate drinks per day can sabotage an otherwise healthy diet. If you enjoy the taste and fizz in sodas, try switching to diet sodas or sparkling water. It makes a big difference. Most diet drinks contain zero grams of carbohydrate because they're sweetened with low-calorie sweeteners, so they won't raise your blood glucose.

Many people think that fruit drinks and juices are healthy drink choices, but they can contain a lot of carbohydrate and calories as well. If you want to drink a glass of fruit juice now and then, watch your portion size. Or, if you're craving fruit juice, try a glass of water flavored with a squeeze of lemon or lime juice instead. You may also be able to curb your craving with a fresh piece of fruit. Fruits still contain calories and carbohydrates, but whole fruits have fiber that fruit juices don't provide. Your best bet is to chew your fruit instead of drinking it.

Choosing the best drinks

When it comes to drinks, try to stick to zero-calorie or very low-calorie drinks, including the following:

>> Water

>> Unsweetened tea (black, green, herbal)

>> Black coffee

>> Diet soda

>> Other low-calorie drinks/drink mixes (look for options with less than 10 calories and 5 grams of carbohydrate per serving)

Is alcohol off limits?

You may be surprised to read that alcohol is not off limits for people with diabetes. But moderation is key when drinking alcoholic beverages. Women should have no more than one drink per day, and men should have no more than two drinks per day. One drink equals 12 ounces of beer, 5 ounces of wine, or 1½ ounces of distilled spirits.

TIP

Enjoy alcohol safely, especially when you have diabetes. A few easy tips and tricks can help you stay safe:

>> Don't drink on an empty stomach or replace foods in your regular meal plan with alcohol. Alcohol can lower your blood glucose level, and drinking on an empty stomach may cause you to become intoxicated more quickly. So it's a good idea to have food with your alcoholic drink.

>> When you're drinking a mixed drink, choose calorie-free mixers like diet sodas or diet tonic water to avoid extra calories and carbohydrates that will make it harder to manage your blood glucose.

>> Alcohol can lower your blood glucose level (sometime to a dangerously low level), and the symptoms of low blood glucose are very similar to and may be mistaken for the effects of alcohol. For example, both low blood glucose and intoxication can cause dizziness and confusion, hunger and nausea, fatigue and sleepiness, irritability, and other symptoms; this can make it difficult to realize if a person who has been drinking is experiencing low blood glucose. It's important for people with diabetes, especially those who use insulin, to know the symptoms of low blood glucose before leaving home and have a plan to treat lows (this should be discussed this with a healthcare provider). It's also a good idea to wear medical/diabetes identification when drinking.

>> Never drink and drive!

Chapter **2**

Stocking Your Pantry

Building a pantry of nutritious foods and staple ingredients is an important part of healthy eating and makes home cooking easier and more convenient. Keeping healthy ingredients on hand makes it easier to prepare a quick and healthy meal on even the busiest of nights.

In this chapter, we walk you through taking inventory of your kitchen and stocking your pantry with healthy ingredients. In the pages ahead, you'll find lists of staple ingredients that you'll want to keep stocked in your pantry and refrigerator. Along the way, we share a few shopping and food storage tips to help you get the most out of the fresh, canned, and dry ingredients you buy.

Getting Started: Taking Inventory

The first step to building a healthy pantry is to take inventory of the tools and ingredients you already have. You don't want to waste time shopping for ingredients that you already have in your kitchen; for example, you probably don't need to buy a new bottle of olive oil if you already have a half of a bottle left from your last shopping trip. Going through your pantry, refrigerator, and cabinets is a great way to gauge which ingredients, cookware, and utensils you're missing or need to replace on your next trip to the supermarket. This is also a great time to clean out your kitchen and get rid of any ingredients that are past their prime so you can get a fresh start.

Kitchen tools and cookware

If your goal is to cook more healthy meals at home, having the kitchen tools you'll need is a great start. Home cooking doesn't require a lot of expensive tools or gadgets or cookware, but having the basics will help. Here's a list of a few common kitchen tools to keep on hand:

>> Cutting boards

>> Hand-held electric mixer

>> Knives — a paring knife, a serrated knife, and a chef's knife

>> Measuring cups and spoons

>> Meat thermometer (optional)

>> Nonstick pots and pans of various sizes with lids

>> Set of mixing bowls

>> Spoons (slotted, wooden, and metal), spatulas/rubber scrapers, and a wire whisk

>> Strainer/colander

>> Vegetable peeler, cheese grater, can opener

Cleaning out your kitchen

As you're going through your pantry, cabinets, and refrigerator taking inventory, it's a good idea to get rid of any ingredients that are spoiled or that you don't want to keep in the house anymore. Leftover takeout from last weekend, an open carton of milk from a few weeks ago, the spices that have been sitting in your cabinet for several years — all of these things can go in the trash. This will help you de-clutter your refrigerator and pantry, and make room for new healthy items.

In addition to throwing out old or spoiled foods, it may also be helpful to get rid of any high-calorie (or high-fat/high-sugar) foods that you know you'll be tempted to overeat, or at least move them somewhere out of sight. This doesn't mean you have to get rid of every piece of junk food you have in your home; if you can limit your consumption of less healthy foods and only eat them on occasion, that's great. But many people find that they have more success with healthy eating when they stock up on healthy foods and limit junk foods.

TIP

It's important to take inventory and clean out your kitchen before you stock your pantry with healthy foods for the first time, but it's also a good idea to do a mini inventory before each trip to the grocery store. You don't have to do a thorough review of your entire kitchen, just quickly check your pantry and fridge for any important ingredients that you're running low on, and throw away any expired foods. Checking your pantry before shopping will save you time and money at the grocery store!

TIP

As you're cleaning out your kitchen, pay attention to which foods you're getting rid of. Food waste is a concern for many people. If you notice that you're not finishing certain foods before they go bad, note that on your shopping list and consider buying less of those items next time you're at the store or look to see if there is a canned or frozen option available that can be stored longer.

Stocking Up on the Essentials

When you've finished taking inventory of your kitchen, it's time to stock up on diabetes-friendly ingredients! There are several healthy foods and staple ingredients you'll want to keep in your pantry and refrigerator so you're always prepared to make a healthy meal.

Pantry staples

Let's start with staple ingredients that you can keep in your pantry. These are shelf-stable foods and condiments that you can store at room temperature in your pantry for several weeks to several months.

Oils and condiments

Oils, vinegars, and other condiments should be stored in a cool, dry place. Many oils can last months in your pantry if they're opened, and you may be able to store oils even longer in the refrigerator. Check the label of your oils for storage information. If an oil develops an unpleasant smell or taste, it may be time to replace it; oils do go bad after a while. Vinegars have a long shelf life, so you won't have to replace them nearly as often. Here are a few condiments you'll want to stock in your pantry:

>> Canola or vegetable oil

>> Nonstick cooking spray

>> Extra-virgin olive oil

>> Hot sauce (or hot pepper sauce)

>> Low-sodium broth (chicken or vegetable)

>> Reduced-sodium soy sauce

>> Vinegars (white, apple cider, malt, white wine, red wine, balsamic)

>> Worcestershire sauce

Dried herbs and spices

A good collection of herbs and spices is essential when you're cooking healthy meals at home. They're a great way to add flavor to your dishes without adding a lot of extra fat or sodium. Most dried herbs and ground or whole spices are very low in sodium. However, if you purchase premade seasoning blends, check the sodium content. It's a good idea to look for salt-free spices and spice blends options.

Many people think that herbs and spices can be stored in the pantry indefinitely, but the truth is that they start to lose potency and flavor after about 6 months to 1 year. So it's a good idea to purchase these products in small amounts and discard and replace any unused spices at least once a year.

The types of herbs and spices you buy will depend on your personal flavor preferences, but these are some good basic products to keep on hand:

>> Basil

>> Black peppercorns or ground pepper

>> Chili powder

>> Cinnamon

>> Coriander

>> Crushed red pepper

>> Cumin

>> Garlic powder

>> Ginger

>> Mustard powder

>> Nutmeg

>> Oregano

>> Paprika

>> Rosemary

>> Sage

>> Salt

>> Thyme

Sweeteners and baking supplies

It's a common misconception that baked goods are off-limits for people with diabetes. But that's not the case! People with diabetes can still enjoy fluffy pancakes and delicious desserts once in a while. So keep some baking supplies in your pantry for when you try some of the healthy dessert recipes in this book!

What's the deal with sugar substitutes (sometimes called artificial sweeteners or nonnutritive sweeteners)? You may have heard that people with diabetes need to use sugar substitutes in their foods and drinks instead of sugar. People with diabetes can still enjoy foods and beverages sweetened with sugar and other calorie-containing sweeteners as long as they work them into their meal plan (though it's best to enjoy these kinds of foods and drinks in moderation). But sugar substitutes can be a safe option for reducing the amount of calories and carbohydrate in your foods and drinks.

Currently, the U.S. Food and Drug Administration has approved six artificial sweeteners for consumption: acesulfame potassium (or acesulfame K), advantame, aspartame, saccharin, sucralose, and neotame. You'll find these sweeteners on your grocery store shelves under their various brand names. You can add these to your coffee or tea or use them as a table-top sweetener. Some of these sweeteners also come in granular versions that can be used for cooking and baking, and you'll find that many of the dessert recipes in this book call for granulated sugar or brown sugar substitute.

TIP

If you have a recipe that calls for sugar or brown sugar and you decide to use sugar substitutes instead, there are a few things to keep in mind. Baked goods made with sugar substitutes may be lighter in color and lower in volume than those made with sugar. Sugar substitutes can also slightly alter the texture, cooking time, and (in some cases) the taste of baked goods. Read the package instructions carefully for the best way to incorporate the sugar substitute into your recipe.

Here are a few sweeteners and baking supplies to keep in your pantry for those days when you're craving something sweet:

>> Artificial sweetener packets (optional)

>> Baking powder

>> Baking soda

>> Brown sugar

>> Brown sugar substitute

>> Cocoa powder

>> Cornstarch

>> Evaporated milk (fat-free)

>> Flour

>> Sugar

>> Sugar substitute (granulated)

>> Vanilla extract

>> Whole-wheat flour

REMEMBER

Just because a food is made using sugar substitutes doesn't mean it's calorie or carbohydrate free. If you make a batch of cookies with sugar substitute, this may reduce the amount of calories and carbohydrate in the cookies, but other ingredients such as flour and chocolate chips will still contain calories and carbohydrate. You'll still need to account for these foods in your meal plan.

Grains

Whole grains are a better starch choice for people with diabetes because they contain more fiber, vitamins, and minerals than most refined starches. They're great as part of a hearty breakfast or a side dish and make a wonderful addition to salads and soups. Keep a few of these grains on hand; they should stay fresh in your pantry for a few months in a sealed container:

>> Brown or wild rice

>> Farro

>> Millet

>> Oats or oatmeal

>> Quinoa

>> Sorghum

>> Whole-wheat pasta

Canned and dry foods

Beans, peas, and lentils are great additions to any healthy dinner. Although they contain carbohydrate, they're also a source of protein, fiber, and vitamins and minerals. Beans and legumes can be enjoyed as a healthy starch, or a plant-based protein. Stock your shelves with a few different kinds of canned and dried beans. Dried beans can last at least a year in your pantry, especially if stored in an airtight container.

Fresh or frozen vegetables often contain little or no sodium, but canned vegetables have the advantage of being shelf-stable and ready any time you need them. Canned products can have a lot of sodium, so look for low-sodium or no-salt-added varieties of canned beans and vegetables or drain and rinse the canned food before cooking. Canned beans and vegetables usually cook much faster than their fresh or dried counterparts.

The specific types of fruits, vegetables, beans, and legumes you buy will depend on your individual tastes, but here is a list of a few basic canned and dry products to get you started:

» Black beans (canned or dry)

» Canned diced and/or crushed tomatoes

» Canned fruits (packed in water or juice)

» Canned vegetables (low-sodium)

» Cannellini beans (canned or dry)

» Chickpeas (canned or dry)

» Kidney beans (canned or dry)

» Lentils

» Navy beans (canned or dry)

» Nuts or nut spreads (any variety)

» Tomato paste

» Tomato purée

Fresh staples

You'll want to keep a few fresh staple ingredients stocked in your refrigerator. These are the ingredients that you'll use often to add flavor to your meals. For example, many recipes call for garlic, onion, or fresh herbs, so it's a good idea to have these ingredients available. Fresh staples to consider include

» Celery

» Chives

» Cilantro

» Dijon mustard

» Dill

» Eggs or egg substitute

» Fat-free plain yogurt

» Garlic

- » Ginger
- » Lemons and limes
- » Low-fat mayonnaise
- » Low-fat cheese
- » Milk (fat-free)
- » Onions (white or yellow)
- » Parsley
- » Red onions
- » Tomatoes
- » Whole-grain mustard

TIP

In addition to these items, keep frozen versions of a few of your favorite fruits and vegetables in your freezer. That way, even if you can't get to the store, you'll always have some produce handy. And it won't go bad as quickly as fresh produce does! Frozen produce that is stored properly will be safe to eat indefinitely, but the food may begin to lose flavor and quality after a year or two. Enjoy frozen foods by the "best by" date for the best flavor.

Making the Most of Your Pantry

Once you've stocked your pantry and refrigerator, all you'll need to buy at the grocery store is fresh or frozen produce, meat, poultry, and seafood; any snack or specialty items you and your family want; and any staple ingredients that you're running low on. One good strategy for keeping track of your staple ingredients is to keep a running grocery list on your refrigerator or in your smartphone. Every time you run out of an important item, immediately write it on the list so you don't forget to replace it.

If you use a lot of recipes, it can help to pick out your recipes for the week before you go grocery shopping. That way you can read the ingredient lists in the recipes and check your refrigerator and pantry to make sure you have everything you need. Any ingredients that you don't have on hand or don't normally purchase should be added to your shopping list. A little advanced planning can save you some time throughout the week; you won't have to run out to the store for one or two items every time you try a new recipe.

Filling your pantry and refrigerator with healthy ingredients may seem like a lot of work, but it will pay off in the long run. Healthy eating and cooking are easy if you're prepared with some nutritious foods stocked in your kitchen!

Chapter **3**

Making It Healthy: Tips and Techniques

When people are diagnosed with type 2 diabetes, they're often asked to make lifestyle changes to help them manage their blood glucose levels and prevent or delay the complications of diabetes. But changing your eating habits can be a daunting task, especially if you're just learning how to eat well with diabetes. Luckily, you don't need to transform your diet overnight. You can make small changes to your cooking and eating habits to improve the quality of your diet and help you enjoy your time in the kitchen! In this chapter, we offer some simple tips and techniques that will help you on your path toward healthy eating success.

TIP

A good first step when learning how to eat healthy with diabetes is to meet with a registered dietitian (RD) or registered dietitian nutritionist (RDN) who will sit down with you to help you create an individualized meal plan based on your personal eating patterns and food preferences that will help you manage your blood glucose and reach your personal diabetes goals. The tips and techniques discussed in this chapter are meant to help you embrace healthy eating and cooking in the hopes that changing your eating habits doesn't have to be difficult or stressful. However, the information in this chapter is not a substitute for a consultation with an RD or RDN or an individualized meal plan.

This chapter not only shows you easy ways to make your meals healthier, but also helps you maintain the joy of eating as you make changes to your diet. Healthy eating begins in the mind. Adjusting how you think about food is often a big step toward healthier living. The tips in this chapter will address four main aspects of healthy eating: choosing ingredients, using healthy cooking techniques, understanding your appetite, and creating a positive mind-set. Adopting a few healthy techniques in each of these areas will prepare you to make any recipe or meal healthy!

REMEMBER

You don't need to make a lot of changes all at once. Trying out just a few healthy eating tips each week can go a long way when it comes to improving your diet and managing your blood glucose.

Now let's take a closer look at some of the tips and techniques you can use in your kitchen to help you eat well and enjoy every minute of it.

It's All about Ingredients

Healthy, quality ingredients are the foundation of a nutritious meal. But it's not always easy to know which ingredients are the healthiest options, and it can be tempting when shopping and cooking to select less healthy ingredients. This section gives you simple tips to help you avoid temptation while shopping and find the best ingredients for your meals. If you're not sure what kinds of foods people with diabetes can eat, visit Chapter 1 for detailed information on the best food choices for people with diabetes. Or you can meet with an RD or RDN to discuss the best food choices for you. It's a good idea to have a grasp of this information before you begin shopping.

REMEMBER

Generally speaking, good food choices for people with diabetes include

>> Fresh, canned, or frozen fruits and nonstarchy vegetables (including tomatoes, carrots, broccoli, asparagus, onions, peppers, salad greens, and many more)

>> Lean sources of protein

>> Whole-grains and starchy vegetables (such as potatoes, corn, green peas, and winter squash)

>> "Healthy" unsaturated fats (such as plant oils, nuts, and seeds)

When shopping, try to select these foods instead of processed, high-fat, and high-sodium or high-sugar foods.

In this section, we also look at some easy ingredient substitutions you can use to make some of your favorite recipes a little more diabetes-friendly. Making a few simple changes to the ingredient list of a recipe can significantly reduce the amount of fat, sodium, and carbohydrate in a dish.

Shop wisely

TIP

The idea of shopping for healthy ingredients may seem intimidating, but we have a few straightforward tips to help you make the most of your next trip to the grocery store and take the stress out of shopping:

» **Don't shop when you're hungry.** Shopping when you're hungry can lower your resolve to choose healthy ingredients. If you're hungry, you may reach for comfort foods or snacks that contain a lot of carbohydrate, fat, sodium, or sugar instead of looking for more nutritious choices. Or you may end up buying more food than you actually need. Eat a healthy snack before shopping if it's been a while since your last meal.

» **Bring a shopping list.** This seems like an obvious tip, but it can make a big difference! Bring a complete shopping list with you and try to stick to it. If you focus on finding the healthy ingredients you need, you'll be less tempted to buy foods you don't need. Don't forget to check your refrigerator and pantry before you go shopping; if you're out of any staple ingredients (spices, herbs, condiments, eggs, milk), add them to your list.

» **Avoid the center aisles of the grocery store.** When you get to the grocery store, take a moment to plan your route through the store. Stick to shopping on the outer perimeter of the store if possible; this is where you'll find fresh produce and other fresh ingredients. The center aisles hold processed foods. You may need to dip into a few aisles to grab an item or two, but it's best to do most of your shopping in the outer sections of the store.

» **Skip "sugar-free" or "diabetic" foods.** You'll see many products in the grocery store that are labeled "sugar-free" or marketed to people with diabetes. You do not need to purchase these foods. They're often expensive, and some of these products (such as sugar-free cookies or candies) contain sugar alcohols that may cause gastrointestinal discomfort if eaten in large amounts. You're better off choosing fresh, whole ingredients than "diabetic" foods.

» **Keep an eye on sodium and sugar.** When it comes to produce, purchasing fresh or frozen unprocessed ingredients as often as possible is the ideal. Canned fruits and vegetables are also good options, but keep an eye on the sodium and sugar content of these products. Look for low-sodium canned vegetables or vegetable juices. If you can't find low-sodium canned vegetables, drain and rinse these foods before using them. Fruits canned in juice or extra-light syrup are the best options when it comes to fruit.

>> **Add some variety to your diet.** Choose a wide range of colors of fruits and vegetables from the grocery store. Eating all different colors and kinds of produce will ensure you get a full spectrum of vitamins, minerals, and other beneficial nutrients in your diet. Add some variety to your whole-grain choices as well; instead of sticking with brown rice, try adding quinoa, farro, barley, or bulgur wheat to your shopping cart.

>> **Read food labels.** When buying packaged products, take a look at the Nutrition Facts panels and compare nutrients for similar foods to find the one that will work best with your meal plan.

Ingredient swaps for healthier recipes

One of the reasons people find it so overwhelming to make healthy food choices is because they have the idea that eating healthier means giving up all of the foods they love. Well, don't worry — you don't have to throw away grandma's potato salad recipe or stop cooking your favorite casserole just because you have diabetes!

The trick is to find little ways to make these foods healthier or eat smaller portions. You may be able to reduce the carbohydrate, fat, sodium, and/or calorie content of your favorite recipes to help them better fit into your diabetes meal plan. Swapping out a few of the less healthy ingredients in a recipe for more nutritious options can make all the difference. Try some of the common ingredient substitutions shown in Table 3-1.

TABLE 3-1   **Ingredient Substitutions**

Instead of . . .	Try . . .
All-purpose flour	Whole-wheat flour (this may affect the texture of baked goods)
Bacon	Reduced-sodium Canadian bacon, turkey bacon, or smoked turkey slices
Butter (for sautéing)	Vegetable oil, olive oil, or any other plant oil
Deli meat	Grilled or baked chicken or turkey breast
Full-fat cheese	Reduced-fat cheese (or choose a full-fat cheese with a stronger flavor and reduce the amount used)
Full-fat yogurt	Nonfat yogurt
Ground beef	Very lean ground beef, ground chicken or turkey, or replace some of the beef with beans or lentils
Hamburger buns	Whole-wheat buns or roasted portobello mushrooms

Instead of . . .	Try . . .
Hash browns	Grated zucchini
Mashed potatoes	Cauliflower mash
Mayonnaise	Light mayonnaise, mustard, or mashed avocado
Salt	Decrease the amount of salt or use herbs, spices, and salt-free seasoning blends to add more flavor
Sour cream	Plain nonfat yogurt (regular or Greek)
Sugar (for baking)	Replace some or all of the sugar with granulated artificial sweetener or artificial sweetener baking blend (follow package instructions)
Tortillas (for tacos)	Whole-wheat tortillas or large lettuce or kale leaves
White bread	100 percent whole-wheat bread
White pasta	Whole-wheat pasta, spaghetti squash, or zucchini ribbons
White rice	Brown rice, wild rice, or another whole grain
Whole eggs	Egg whites or egg substitute
Whole or 2 percent milk	Fat-free or 1 percent milk

You can use these ingredient swaps in just about any recipe! Keep in mind that you don't need to find a healthier substitute for every ingredient in a recipe. Even one or two ingredient swaps can make a dish healthier. A good place to start is finding a healthier option to replace the ingredient that is highest in fat, sodium, or carbohydrate.

WARNING

Swapping ingredients when baking can change the look and texture of baked goods. It may take some trial and error to figure out which healthy ingredient swaps work best in your favorite baked-good recipe. If you decide to use a sugar substitute in your recipe, read the tips on the package so you know how much of the sugar substitute to use.

TIP

Another great way to make your recipes and meals healthier is to use some non-starchy vegetables to add bulk to a dish or balance out your plate. Because non-starchy vegetables are low in calories and carbohydrate, you can enjoy these vegetables in larger amounts than other foods, making them a great food option when you want to satisfy your hunger without compromising your meal plan. Here are a few simple tips for using nonstarchy vegetables to your advantage:

>> **Bulk it up.** Nonstarchy vegetables can provide substance and flavor while adding healthy nutrients and very few calories to a recipe. Add an extra serving of nonstarchy vegetables into your meal by adding them to an omelet

or a pasta dish (the bulk from the veggies may help you eat less pasta). Even if you're not a big fan of vegetables, you can sneak in a serving by finely chopping some vegetables and "hiding" them in a pasta sauce or soup.

>> **Replace some protein with vegetables.** You may be able to slightly reduce the fat and calorie content of a recipe and increase the fiber content by replacing some or all of the meat, seafood, or poultry in a dish with non-starchy vegetables. This works especially well in recipes for combination foods such as soups, casseroles, pasta dishes, or even pizzas. These dishes have so many different ingredients that you may not even notice if you replace half of the animal protein with vegetables!

>> **Pay attention to sides.** If you're cooking a main dish that is a little higher in fat, carbohydrate, or sodium than you would like, pair it with healthier side dishes so you have a balanced meal. For example, if you're cooking a burger for dinner, maybe opt for a side salad or a nonstarchy vegetable like baked zucchini wedges instead of making french fries.

Adjusting Your Cooking Habits

Before you were diagnosed with diabetes, you may have prepared your meals without giving a lot of thought to the method (frying, baking, or grilling) you used. Maybe you used whatever fat was handy to sauté vegetables and weren't worried about a food's fat content. You just wanted to cook something quickly and eat it so you could get back to your busy day.

A diabetes diagnosis requires you to monitor your health more closely. Now you may need to put more thought into how you prepare dishes. Would you be better off eating a chicken breast that's been fried or grilled? How can you cut some fat from your diet? Can you find a way to take those veggies from bland to whiz-bang delicious? We help you find the answers to these questions in the following sections.

Focusing on technique

Although it's true that healthy ingredients are the basis for a healthy dish, it's also important to use cooking methods that bring out the flavor of these ingredients without compromising their nutritional value. When it comes to cooking, some methods are better than others. Deep frying or adding lots of fat and salt to foods, for example, can turn healthy ingredients into an unhealthy dish and contribute many grams of fat and sodium to your meal. But using healthy cooking preparations doesn't mean you have to eat plain baked proteins and steamed vegetables.

Consider the following healthy cooking methods that will keep your meal plan on track without sacrificing taste:

» **Sautéing:** Sautéing refers to frying ingredients in a pan using a little fat. Depending on the type and amount of fat used, this can be a relatively healthy cooking method. Try to avoid sautéing your foods in animal fats like butter; instead use a small amount (aim for 1 tablespoon or less) of a vegetable oil such as olive oil, canola oil, or avocado oil. Use nonstick cookware when sautéing ingredients, or spray the pan with nonstick vegetable oil spray so you don't need to use as much oil. You can also try sautéing foods in a small amount of cooking wine, broth, or water if you don't want to use oil.

» **Stir-frying:** Stir-frying is a method similar to sautéing in which ingredients are fried in a small amount of very hot oil. Certain oils are more appropriate for high-heat cooking methods (like stir-frying) than others; use an oil with a high smoke point, such as avocado, canola, safflower, or peanut oil. Heating an oil with a low smoke point too far beyond that smoke point could possibly cause a fire. It's important to stir continuously when preparing a stir-fry. You should use a plant-based oil for stir-frying instead of using butter.

» **Boiling and poaching:** Boiling and poaching are both healthy cooking methods because they don't require adding fats to your ingredients. In both of these methods, the ingredients are cooking in hot liquid (usually water). Boiling is a good way to prepare starchy and nonstarchy vegetables such as potatoes, corn, dried beans, carrots, and broccoli. Poaching is a slightly gentler method of cooking that is great for preparing eggs, fish, and vegetables.

» **Steaming:** Steaming fish, vegetables, and even some grains is another healthy cooking method because no added fat is required to cook the ingredients. Instead the steam from boiling water gently cooks the ingredients, keeping them moist.

» **Roasting, grilling, or broiling:** All three of these cooking methods can be healthy ways to prepare meat, poultry, and seafood. Try not to add a lot of extra fats to ingredients before cooking. And if you're basting meat or poultry, try using a small amount of broth instead of basting with the pan drippings. Roasting or grilling vegetables (and fruits if you're feeling adventurous) is a wonderful way to enhance their flavor. Broiling, however, has the potential to dry out vegetables quickly.

» **Microwaving:** Almost everyone has a microwave, though few people associate microwaving with healthy eating. But the microwave can be a big asset to a healthy kitchen because it saves you time and you can cook many ingredients in the microwave without adding fat. Use your microwave to cook vegetables or bake a potato so you don't have to turn on the stove or oven. Many grocery stores even sell frozen vegetables that steam in the bag or microwavable rice.

You can take advantage of all these different cooking methods when you're preparing diabetes-friendly meals! Just remember to keep the amount of fat used while cooking to a minimum, and choose vegetable oils (sources of unsaturated fat) over animal fats such as butter and lard.

Reducing the amount of fat you add to dishes

Reducing the amount of oil you use while cooking is a great way to make sure you're not adding too much fat to your foods. Excess fat can cause weight gain, and eating too much saturated fat (found in butter, lard, cream, poultry skin, full-fat dairy products, and other animal fats) can increase your risk for heart disease. People with diabetes already have an increased risk of heart complications, so it's important to monitor your fat intake.

TIP

Here are a few easy ways to reduce the amount of fat in your meals:

» If you're pan-frying meat, drain the fat off the meat as you're cooking.

» After making a soup or stew, let it cool to room temperature and then chill it in the refrigerator until the fat settles at the top of the soup and hardens. Skim the fat off the top and discard it before reheating and enjoying the soup.

» If you're roasting, grilling, or broiling meat, cook it on a rack so the fat can drain off the meat as it cooks.

» Remove the skin from chicken, turkey, and other poultry either before cooking or before eating. The skin contains saturated fat.

» Avoid recipes and foods with butter- or cream-based sauces.

Amping up the flavor

People with diabetes need to find healthy ways to flavor their foods without adding high-fat or high-sodium ingredients to the mix. Here are a few cooking tips to help you boost the flavor of your foods:

» **Marinate your proteins.** Try marinating meats, poultry, and seafood using fresh herbs, spices, lemon or lime juice, cooking wine, vinegar, or low-sodium broth. These ingredients are low in fat, sodium, and calories and are a healthier alternative to store-bought marinades. You can marinate your vegetables, too!

>> **Use herbs and spices.** Adding fresh or dried herbs, ground spices, or salt-free spice blends to a dish is a great way to add flavor without adding salt or fat. Experiment with fresh herbs — such as dill, parsley, cilantro, sage, rosemary, and thyme — to find out which flavor combinations are your favorites. If you're using dried herbs and spices, make sure they haven't been sitting in your spice cabinet for too long; many bottled herbs and spices begin to lose potency after 6 months to 1 year.

Be careful not to overseason your dish. Add herbs and spices in small quantities at first and taste the food to see if you need more flavor.

>> **Cook with aromatic vegetables.** Aromatic vegetables, such as garlic, ginger, onion, and celery add a wonderful smell and incredible flavor to a dish. You'll be amazed at what adding some aromatic vegetables to a stir-fry, soup stock, or roasting pan (along with a protein or other vegetables) can do to enhance the taste of an otherwise plain dish. It's a good idea to always keep a few of these vegetables on hand in your kitchen.

>> **Add some citrus.** The juice of citrus fruits is a great way to add brightness to a dish and enhance its natural flavors without adding salt. Try adding a squeeze of fresh lemon, lime, or even orange juice to fish, vegetables, or grains either before or after cooking. Citrus juice also tastes great in marinades and salad dressings.

Eating Less

In addition to making healthier food choices, many people with diabetes need to adjust their eating habits so they eat less food. Eating too many servings of a food, even a healthy food, will affect your blood glucose and can add to weight gain. Eating the right serving sizes for your calorie goals and practicing portion control are essential parts of any healthy eating plan.

If you find yourself struggling to control your appetite, the following tips may help:

>> **Avoid skipping meals.** The hunger caused by missing a meal can lead you to overeat later in the day and cause your blood glucose to rise or fall.

>> **Remove distractions while eating so you can recognize when your body is full.**

>> **To make sure you're not serving yourself too much, measure out the correct serving sizes for your foods instead of estimating for a while to become familiar with the serving sizes that are right for you.**

>> **Try serving your foods and beverage in smaller dishes and cups.** It sounds a little silly, but using smaller dishes can make regular portions of foods and drinks look larger. It can help trick your mind into thinking you're eating more.

>> **If you have favorite junk foods that you crave, you don't have to deny yourself these foods.** Denying yourself may backfire and make you want them even more, causing you to overindulge! You can eat these foods in small portions sometimes as long as you account for them in your meal plan. This means counting the amount of calories and/or carbohydrate in these foods toward you daily or mealtime goal (if you're tracking calories or carbohydrate) or forgoing other starchy or high-calorie foods during the meal and pairing the food you're craving with healthy foods, such as nonstarchy vegetables or lean protein.

>> **If you just ate but still feel hungry, take a moment to examine your emotions.** Are you bored, stressed, angry, or sad? Some people feel compelled to eat based on their emotions, so it's important to figure out if you're experiencing true hunger or if you're being triggered by your emotions.

>> **If you feel hungry often, try to distract yourself with a couple of different activities.** Before you indulge, try drinking a glass of water, taking a short walk or doing another form of light exercise, or reading or watching TV.

If you were used to eating large portions of food before you were diagnosed with diabetes, appetite control may be a difficult part of transitioning to a healthier lifestyle. Put these tips to good use, and after a few weeks, your appetite should adjust to your new eating habits. For more tips on portion control, see Chapter 17.

TIP

If you can't control your appetite despite your best efforts, discuss this with your doctor, who can give you a referral to a RD or RDN. They can help you make the best food choices, adjust your meal plan to help you avoid hunger, or recommend another form of therapy.

A New Attitude

Eating nutritious meals and increasing your knowledge to make better food choices are both vital parts of a healthy lifestyle. But believe it or not, eating well isn't just about the food — it's also about your attitude. Diabetes can be tough to manage and changing your lifestyle can be stressful, but if you're always focused on the negative aspects of diabetes management, you'll find it harder to take care of yourself.

TIP

To make positive lifestyle changes last, adjust your thinking to embrace your new, healthier habits. Set yourself up for success by following these tips for finding joy in healthy eating and cooking:

>> **Manage your expectations.** Making better food choices and cooking healthy meals aren't skills that you pick up overnight. If you're not familiar with diabetes nutrition or don't have much experience in the kitchen, learning how to do these things can take time. Start by making small changes to the way you shop for ingredients and cook dishes (hopefully the tips in this chapter will help). You also need to manage your expectations when it comes to diabetes and other health goals. For example, if one of your goals is to lose weight, don't expect to lose 10 pounds in 1 week. Set small, realistic goals for yourself, and try not to get discouraged if things aren't progressing as quickly as you'd like.

>> **Gain confidence in the kitchen.** Eating well with diabetes does require some cooking, and this can be intimidating if you're not used to spending much time in the kitchen. Make things easy on yourself by sticking to quick, simple recipes as you're learning. Many of the recipes in this book are great for beginner cooks!

TIP

Read through each recipe carefully and look up any ingredients or cooking terms that you're unfamiliar with. Making mistakes is part of the process, so try not to be too hard on yourself.

>> **Make healthy eating fun.** Eating well doesn't have to be a chore. Find something positive that motivates you to continue eating healthy foods. You might discover as you begin spending time in the kitchen that you really love cooking. If that's the case, that's great! Look for new healthy recipes to try each week, take a cooking class to inspire you, or make nutritious menus to share with your friends and family.

If you're not a fan of cooking, try to include something you love in the process. If you're a music fan, make a playlist to listen to as you cook dinner each night. If you love spending time with your friends, invite them over to help you cook. Fan of the outdoors? Visit your local farmers' market and find fresh ingredients to prepare. Find some aspect of healthy eating that excites you.

>> **Savor your food and slow down.** One of the best ways to maintain a positive attitude about healthy eating is to actually experience and allow yourself to enjoy healthy foods. It can be tough on busy days, but it's important to take a break from everything else when you can and focus on the food you're eating without distractions. Try to appreciate the progress you're making as a cook and the fact that you have nutritious food to eat.

>> **Find a support system.** Maintaining a healthy lifestyle can be tough even if you maintain a positive attitude. Sometime it helps to talk to someone about what you're going through. Is there a friend or family member who is supportive of your health goals and lifestyle changes whom you can turn to? Don't be afraid to talk to that person if you're feeling overwhelmed. Diabetes support groups (both online and in person) are another great resource. If you're struggling with a specific aspect of healthy eating or diabetes management, you can also ask your doctor or dietitian for help.

2
Digging into Main Dishes

Chapter **4**

Breakfasts

RECIPES IN THIS CHAPTER

- **Baked French Toast with Raspberry Sauce**
- **Fresh Blueberry Pancakes**
- **Griddle Corn Cakes**
- **Hash Browns**
- **Italian Frittata**
- **Mini Breakfast Quiches**
- **Turkey Sausage Patties**
- **Western Omelet**

We've all heard that breakfast is the most important meal of the day. But breakfast can also be a difficult meal for people with diabetes. So many traditional breakfast foods — such as breads, sugary pastries, pancakes, bacon, and sausage — are high in carbohydrate and/or fat, two nutrients that people with diabetes need to monitor in their diets. Fortunately, you don't have to give up on hearty French toast, savory sausage, golden hash browns, or other breakfast classics just because you have diabetes. A few simple ingredient changes can go a long way toward making your favorite breakfast dishes diabetes friendly!

The recipes in this chapter swap out some of the less-than-healthy ingredients in breakfast foods for options that are lower in fat or higher in fiber and other nutrients. Using whole-wheat bread instead of white bread or replacing some or all of the white flour in a recipe with whole-wheat flour can make dishes like pancakes and French toast more nutritious. Try substituting lean breakfast meats, such as the Turkey Sausage Patties, and low-fat or fat-free dairy for higher-fat ingredients in your favorite dish. Looking to incorporate veggies into your morning? Savory breakfast recipes like Hash Browns, Italian Frittata, Western Omelet, and other egg dishes are a delicious way to squeeze more nonstarchy vegetables into your meal plan.

People with diabetes can still enjoy a hearty homemade breakfast, especially if they make a few health-conscious adjustments to traditional recipes. This chapter shows you how! So make time for breakfast each morning and start your day off right with these incredible recipes.

Baked French Toast with Raspberry Sauce

PREP TIME: ABOUT 5 MIN PLUS CHILLING TIME	COOK TIME: 30 MIN	SERVINGS: 4	SERVING SIZE: 2 SLICES

INGREDIENTS

1 cup egg substitute

⅔ cup fat-free milk

1 teaspoon cinnamon

½ teaspoon nutmeg

8 slices whole-wheat bread

2 cups frozen or fresh raspberries

1 tablespoon orange juice

1 teaspoon vanilla extract

2 teaspoons cornstarch

DIRECTIONS

1 In a medium bowl, beat together the egg substitute, milk, cinnamon, and nutmeg.

2 In a casserole dish, lay the bread slices side by side. Pour on the egg–milk mixture, cover, and refrigerate overnight.

3 The next day, bake the French toast at 350 degrees for about 30 minutes until golden brown and slightly puffed.

4 To make the raspberry sauce, puree the raspberries in a blender. Strain to remove the seeds.

5 In a small saucepan, combine the pureed berries with the orange juice, vanilla, and cornstarch. Bring to a boil and cook for 1 minute until the mixture is thickened. Serve over French toast.

PER SERVING: *Choices/Exchanges: 2 Starch, ½ Fruit, 1 Lean Protein; Calories 230 (from Fat 20); Fat 2.5g (Saturated 0.5g, Trans 0.0g); Cholesterol 0mg; Sodium 390mg; Potassium 400mg; Total Carbohydrate 37g (Dietary Fiber 8g; Sugars 8g); Protein 15g; Phosphorus 190mg.*

Fresh Blueberry Pancakes

PREP TIME: ABOUT 5 MIN	COOK TIME: 10 MIN	SERVINGS: 8	SERVING SIZE: TWO 4-INCH PANCAKES

INGREDIENTS

1 cup whole-wheat flour

1½ teaspoon baking powder

Zest of 1 lemon

1 teaspoon cinnamon

1 egg white

¾ cup low-fat buttermilk

¼ cup fat-free vanilla yogurt

1 tablespoon canola oil

½ cup fresh blueberries, washed and drained

DIRECTION

1 In a medium bowl, combine the flour, baking powder, lemon zest, and cinnamon; set aside.

2 In a small bowl, combine the egg white, buttermilk, yogurt, and oil, and mix well. Add the wet mixture to the dry ingredients, stirring until moistened. Then gently fold in the blueberries.

3 Coat a griddle or skillet with cooking spray. Pour 2 tablespoons of batter for each pancake onto a hot griddle. Turn the pancakes when the tops are covered with tiny bubbles and the edges are golden brown.

PER SERVING: *Choices/Exchanges: 1 Starch, ½ Fat; Calories 90 (from Fat 20); Fat 2.5g (Saturated 0.3g, Trans 0.0g); Cholesterol 0mg; Sodium 105mg; Potassium 120mg; Total Carbohydrate 14g (Dietary Fiber 2g; Sugars 3g); Protein 4g; Phosphorus 165mg.*

Griddle Corn Cakes

PREP TIME: ABOUT 5 MIN	COOK TIME: 10 MIN	SERVINGS: 6	SERVING SIZE: 2 PANCAKES

INGREDIENTS

1 cup whole-wheat flour

2 teaspoons baking powder

1 tablespoon fructose

¾ cup low-fat buttermilk

1 egg white

2 tablespoons canola oil

1 cup corn kernels (frozen or fresh; if frozen, defrost)

DIRECTIONS

1 In a medium bowl, combine the flour, baking powder, and fructose.

2 In another bowl, combine the buttermilk, egg white, and oil. Stir in the corn kernels. Slowly add the wet mixture to the dry ingredients, just to blend. A few lumps will remain.

3 On a heated nonstick griddle, pour ¼ cup batter per cake. Cook cakes for about 3 minutes, flip them over, and cook 1–2 minutes more, until golden brown. Serve.

PER SERVING: *Choices/Exchanges: 1½ Starch, 1 Fat; Calories 150 (from Fat 50); Fat 6.0g (Saturated 0.6g, Trans 0.0g); Cholesterol 0mg; Sodium 160mg; Potassium 190mg; Total Carbohydrate 23g (Dietary Fiber 3g; Sugars 4g); Protein 5g, Phosphorus 270mg.*

Hash Browns

PREP TIME: ABOUT 5 MIN | COOK TIME: 10 MIN | SERVINGS: 4 | SERVING SIZE: ½ CUP

INGREDIENTS

2 large baking potatoes (about 10 ounces each), unpeeled

2 tablespoons minced onion

2 tablespoons minced red pepper

2 tablespoons minced green pepper

1 garlic clove, minced

½ teaspoon paprika

⅓ teaspoon salt

⅛ teaspoon freshly ground black pepper

¼ teaspoon finely chopped fresh baby dill

DIRECTIONS

1 With a hand grater or a food processor with grater attachment, shred each potato. In a large bowl, combine the potatoes with the remaining ingredients.

2 Coat a large skillet with cooking spray and place over medium heat until hot.

3 Pack the potato mixture firmly into the skillet; cook for 6–8 minutes or until the bottom is browned. Invert the potato patty onto a plate and return to the skillet, cooked side up.

4 Continue cooking over medium heat for another 6–8 minutes until the bottom is browned. Remove from heat and cut into 4 wedges.

PER SERVING: *Choices/Exchanges: 1½ Starch; Calories 110 (from Fat 0); Fat 0.0g (Saturated 0.0g, Trans 0.0g); Cholesterol 0mg; Sodium 200mg; Potassium 590mg; Total Carbohydrate 24g (Dietary Fiber 3g; Sugars 2g); Protein 3g; Phosphorus 80mg.*

Italian Frittata

INGREDIENTS

2 tablespoons extra-virgin olive oil

2 medium yellow onions, sliced thinly

6 large eggs, beaten until foamy

2 cups mixed steamed vegetables (try chopped broccoli, asparagus, and red bell peppers)

2 teaspoons garlic, minced

1 bunch fresh basil, finely chopped

½ teaspoon freshly ground black pepper

¼ cup freshly grated Parmigiano-Reggiano cheese, for garnish

DIRECTIONS

1 Preheat the oven to 350 degrees. Add the oil to a large, wide, ovenproof skillet and heat over medium heat.

2 Add the onions and sauté until lightly golden, approximately 5–10 minutes.

3 In a large bowl, combine the remaining ingredients (except the cheese), and add to the skillet.

4 Place the skillet in the oven and bake the frittata for 14–17 minutes until set. Remove from the oven and loosen the edges with a spatula. Sprinkle with grated cheese, cut into wedges, and serve.

PER SERVING: *Choices/Exchanges: 2 Nonstarchy Vegetable, 1 Medium-Fat Protein, 1 Fat; Calories 160 (from Fat 90); Fat 10.0g (Saturated 2.9g, Trans 0.0g); Cholesterol 190mg; Sodium 105mg; Potassium 340mg; Total Carbohydrate 9g (Dietary Fiber 3g; Sugars 4g); Protein 9g; Phosphorus 175mg.*

Mini Breakfast Quiches

PREP TIME: 10 MIN | COOK TIME: 20 MIN | SERVINGS: 6 | SERVING SIZE: 2 INDIVIDUAL QUICHES

INGREDIENTS

4 ounces diced green chilies

¼ cup diced pimiento

1 small eggplant, cubed

3 cups precooked brown rice

½ cup egg whites

⅓ cup fat-free milk

½ teaspoon cumin

1 bunch fresh cilantro or Italian parsley, finely chopped

1 cup shredded reduced-fat cheddar cheese, divided

DIRECTIONS

1 Preheat the oven to 400 degrees. Spray a 12-cup muffin tin with nonstick cooking spray.

2 In a large mixing bowl, combine all the ingredients except ½ cup of the cheese.

3 Add a dash of salt and pepper, if desired.

4 Spoon the mixture evenly into muffin cups, and sprinkle with the remaining cheese. Bake for 12–15 minutes or until set. Carefully remove the quiches from the pan, arrange on a platter, and serve.

PER SERVING: *Choices/Exchanges: 1½ Starch, 2 Nonstarchy Vegetable, 1 Lean Protein, ½ Fat; Calories 230 (from Fat 45); Fat 5.0g (Saturated 2.7g, Trans 0.0g); Cholesterol 10mg; Sodium 230mg; Potassium 420mg; Total Carbohydrate 35g (Dietary Fiber 4g, Sugars 5g); Protein 12g; Phosphorus 255mg.*

Turkey Sausage Patties

PREP TIME: 10 MIN | COOK TIME: 10 MIN | SERVINGS: 4 | SERVING SIZE: 2 OUNCES

INGREDIENTS

½ pound extra-lean ground turkey breast

2 tablespoons low-sodium beef broth

½ tablespoon lemon juice

2 tablespoons Homemade Seasoned Bread Crumbs (see Chapter 14)

⅛ teaspoon fennel seeds

⅛ teaspoon freshly ground black pepper

⅛ teaspoon ground red pepper

DIRECTIONS

1 In a large bowl, combine all the ingredients; cover, and set aside for at least 15–20 minutes (refrigerate if overnight).

2 Coat a large skillet with cooking spray, and place over medium heat until hot.

3 Shape the mixture into 4 patties, and place in the hot skillet. Fry the patties for 5–6 minutes on each side, remove, and let drain on paper towels.

4 Transfer to a serving platter, and serve while hot.

TIP: Prepare these patties 1 day in advance, and the flavor will be even better the next day.

PER SERVING: *Choices/Exchanges: 2 Lean Protein; Calories 80 (from Fat 15); Fat 1.5g (Saturated 0.3g, Trans 0.0g); Cholesterol 30mg; Sodium 50mg; Potassium 170mg; Total Carbohydrate 1g (Dietary Fiber 0g, Sugars 0g); Protein 15g; Phosphorus 140mg.*

Western Omelet

PREP TIME: ABOUT 5 MIN	COOK TIME: 10 MIN	SERVINGS: 2	SERVING SIZE: ½ OMELET

INGREDIENTS

1½ teaspoons canola oil

¾ cup egg whites

¼ cup minced lean ham

2 tablespoons minced green bell pepper

2 tablespoons minced onion

⅛ teaspoon freshly ground black pepper

DIRECTIONS

1 In a medium nonstick skillet over medium-low heat, heat the oil.

2 In a small mixing bowl, beat the egg whites slightly, and add the remaining ingredients along with a dash of salt, if desired. Pour the egg mixture into the heated skillet.

3 When the omelet begins to set, gently lift the edges of the omelet with a spatula, and tilt the skillet to allow the uncooked portion to flow underneath. Continue cooking until the eggs are firm. Then transfer to a serving platter.

PER SERVING: *Choices/Exchanges: 2 Lean Protein, ½ Fat; Calories 110 (from Fat 40); Fat 4.5g (Saturated 0.6g, Trans 0.0g); Cholesterol 10mg; Sodium 380mg; Potassium 240mg; Total Carbohydrate 2g (Dietary Fiber 0g, Sugars 1g); Protein 15g; Phosphorus 60mg.*

Chapter 5
Soups and Stews

For instant comfort, few things are more effective than a warm bowl of soup. Soups make a great lunch or light dinner. But many canned soups are high in sodium. Luckily, making a healthy, delicious soup from scratch is easier than you think. Many of the recipes in this chapter are good to prepare on busy nights because they require minimal prep and can simmer unattended for a while. And most soups freeze and travel well, so you can keep single portions on hand for an easy weeknight meal or take a serving with you to enjoy at work!

Most important for people with diabetes, homemade soups are a tasty vehicle for incorporating more vegetables, legumes, and lean proteins into your meal plan without a lot of added fat or sodium. The recipes in this chapter use fresh produce and low-sodium products such as broth and canned tomatoes to keep these soups diabetes friendly. But remember: Healthy doesn't mean boring! You'll be surprised by the exciting flavors you'll find in this chapter. Whether you're looking for a heartier dish (like English Beef Stew or Spicy Turkey Chili), or a more delicate, refreshing soup (like Cream of Carrot Soup), there's a recipe for you!

TIP

Got a fridge full of leftovers? Soup recipes are a great way to use the rest of those baby carrots before they go bad, or get rid of that takeout container of brown rice in the fridge. Many of the recipes in this chapter can be varied to use ingredients you have on hand. Just make sure to account for those ingredients in your meal plan.

Comforting Chicken and Mushroom Soup

| PREP TIME: ABOUT 5 MIN | COOK TIME: 20 MIN | SERVINGS: 6 | SERVING SIZE: 1 CUP |

INGREDIENTS

1 quart low-sodium chicken broth

1 tablespoon light soy sauce

1 cup sliced mushrooms, stems removed

1 tablespoon finely chopped scallions

1 tablespoon dry sherry

½ pound boneless, skinless chicken breast, cubed

DIRECTIONS

1 In a stockpot, simmer all ingredients except the chicken for 10 minutes.

2 Add the chicken cubes, and simmer for 6–8 minutes more. Serve with additional soy sauce if desired (but be aware that this will raise the sodium level of the soup).

TIP: Try serving this soup with fresh Buttermilk Biscuits (see Chapter 14).

PER SERVING: *Choices/Exchanges 2 Lean Protein; Calories 70 (from Fat 10); Fat 1g (Saturated 0.2g, Trans 0.0g); Cholesterol 20mg; Sodium 200mg; Potassium 250mg; Total Carbohydrate 1g (Dietary Fiber 0g; Sugars 0g); Protein 13g; Phosphorus 110mg.*

Herbed Chicken Stew with Noodles

PREP TIME: ABOUT 10 MIN	COOK TIME: 40 MIN	SERVINGS: 8	SERVING SIZE: 1 CUP STEW AND ½ CUP NOODLES

INGREDIENTS

1 tablespoon extra-virgin olive oil

1 onion, chopped

2 garlic cloves, minced

1 pound boneless, skinless chicken breast, cubed

2 tablespoons flour

3 cups low-sodium chicken broth

1 cup dry white wine

1 tablespoon chopped fresh thyme (or 1 teaspoon dried)

4 cups cooked egg noodles, hot (from 1/2 pound dry egg noodles)

½ cup minced parsley

DIRECTIONS

1 In a large saucepan, heat the oil and sauté the onion and garlic for about 5 minutes. Add the chicken cubes, and sauté until the chicken is cooked (about 10 minutes).

2 Sprinkle the flour over the chicken. Add the chicken broth, wine, and thyme. Bring to a boil, and then lower the heat and simmer for 30 minutes.

3 Toss together the noodles and the parsley in a large bowl. Pour the stew over the noodles and serve.

TIP: Try using this stew to top rice or a baked potato instead of noodles. Carrots and other root vegetables make a great addition as well.

PER SERVING: *Choices/Exchanges 1½ Starch; 2 Lean Protein; Calories 220 (from Fat 45); Fat 5g (Saturated 1.0g, Trans 0.0g); Cholesterol 55mg; Sodium 85mg; Potassium 270mg; Total Carbohydrate 24g (Dietary Fiber 2g; Sugars 1g); Protein 18g, Phosphorus 185mg.*

Cream of Carrot Soup

PREP TIME: ABOUT 5 MIN	COOK TIME: 15 MIN	SERVINGS: 4	SERVING SIZE: 1 CUP

INGREDIENTS

1 cup plus 2 tablespoons low-sodium chicken broth, divided

3 tablespoons finely chopped shallots or onions

2 tablespoons flour

2 cups fat-free milk, scalded and hot

1 teaspoon cinnamon

1 cup cooked, pureed carrots

Freshly ground black pepper

DIRECTIONS

1 In a stockpot, heat 2 tablespoons of the broth over medium heat. Add the shallots and cook until limp. Sprinkle the shallots with the flour and cook 2–3 minutes.

2 Pour in the hot milk and cook until the mixture thickens. Add the remaining ingredients. Bring almost to a boil, stirring often, and cook for approximately 5 minutes. Add pepper to taste.

VARY IT! Parsnips and sweet potatoes could also be prepared this way.

TIP: This smooth, tasty soup is great to serve for special luncheons.

PER SERVING: *Choices/Exchanges ½ Fat-Free Milk, 1 Nonstarchy Vegetable; Calories 90 (from Fat 0); Fat 0g (Saturated 0.1g, Trans 0.0g); Cholesterol 0mg; Sodium 110mg; Potassium 390mg, Total Carbohydrate 14g (Dietary Fiber 2g; Sugars 9g); Protein 7g; Phosphorus 165mg.*

English Beef Stew

PREP TIME: ABOUT 10 MIN	COOK TIME: 2½ HR	SERVINGS: 8	SERVING SIZE: 1 CUP

INGREDIENTS

2 pounds lean beef for stew, cut into large chunks

1½ tablespoons flour

2 tablespoons canola oil

2 garlic cloves, chopped

2 cups boiling water

1 tablespoon Worcestershire sauce

1⁄16 teaspoon salt

1⁄16 teaspoon freshly ground black pepper

1 large yellow onion, quartered

4 large carrots, peeled and quartered

3 medium potatoes, white or russet, cut into 1-inch cubes

1 cup low-sodium canned stewed tomatoes

DIRECTIONS

1 Roll the beef cubes in the flour. In a large saucepan over medium heat, heat the canola oil. Add the beef, and sauté a few pieces of beef at a time. When all the beef has been browned, add the garlic and stir. Pour the boiling water to the pan.

2 Add the Worcestershire sauce, salt, and pepper. Lower the heat, cover, and let simmer for 1½–2 hours or until the meat is very tender.

3 Add the onion, carrots, potatoes, and tomatoes. Let simmer about 30 minutes until all vegetables are just tender. Transfer to a serving bowl and serve.

PER SERVING: *Choices/Exchanges 1 Starch, 1 Nonstarchy Vegetable, 3 Lean Protein, ½ Fat; Calories 260 (from Fat 70); Fat 8g (Saturated 2.2g, Trans 0.3g); Cholesterol 60mg; Sodium 120mg; Potassium 740mg; Total Carbohydrate 21g (Dietary Fiber 3g; Sugars 5g); Protein 24g; Phosphorus 245mg.*

Fresh Fish Chowder

PREP TIME: ABOUT 10 MIN	COOK TIME: 50 MIN	SERVINGS: 6	SERVING SIZE: 1 CUP

INGREDIENTS

2 tablespoons extra-virgin olive oil

1 large garlic clove, minced

1 small onion, chopped

1 large green bell pepper, chopped

One 14.5-ounce can no-salt-added crushed tomatoes

1 tablespoon tomato paste

½ teaspoon dried basil

½ teaspoon dried oregano

¼ cup dry red wine

$\frac{1}{16}$ teaspoon salt

$\frac{1}{16}$ teaspoon freshly ground black pepper

½ cup uncooked brown rice

½ pound fresh halibut, cubed

2 tablespoons freshly chopped parsley

DIRECTIONS

1 In a 3-quart saucepan, heat the olive oil over medium-high heat. Add the garlic, onion, and green pepper; sauté for 10 minutes over low heat until the vegetables are just tender.

2 Add the tomatoes, tomato paste, basil, oregano, wine, salt, and pepper. Let simmer for 15 minutes. Add the rice and continue to cook for 15 minutes.

3 Add the halibut, and cook for about 5–7 minutes, until the fish is cooked through. Garnish the stew with chopped parsley and serve.

TIP: You can use almost any fish in this chowder — we've used halibut, but cod, mahi mahi, flounder, rockfish, and bass would work well also.

PER SERVING: *Choices/Exchanges 1 Starch, 1 Nonstarchy Vegetable, 1 Lean Protein, 1 Fat; Calories 180 (from Fat 50); Fat 6g (Saturated 0.9g, Trans 0.0g); Cholesterol 10mg; Sodium 75mg; Potassium 540mg; Total Carbohydrate 21g (Dietary Fiber 3g; Sugars 4g); Protein 11g; Phosphorus 170mg.*

Hearty Italian Minestrone

PREP TIME: ABOUT 10 MIN	COOK TIME: 50 MIN	SERVINGS: 8	SERVING SIZE: 1 CUP

INGREDIENTS

½ cup sliced onion

1 tablespoon extra-virgin olive oil

4 cups low-sodium chicken broth

¾ cup diced carrot

½ cup diced potato (with skin)

2 cups sliced cabbage or coarsely chopped spinach

1 cup diced zucchini

½ cup cooked garbanzo beans (drained and rinsed, if canned)

½ cup cooked navy beans (drained and rinsed, if canned)

One 14.5-ounce can low-sodium tomatoes, with liquid

½ cup diced celery

2 tablespoons fresh basil, finely chopped

½ cup uncooked whole-wheat rotini or other shaped pasta

2 tablespoons fresh parsley, finely chopped, for garnish

DIRECTIONS

1 In a large stockpot over medium heat, sauté the onion in oil until the onion is slightly browned. Add the chicken broth, carrot, and potato. Cover and cook over medium heat for 30 minutes.

2 Add the remaining ingredients and cook for an additional 15–20 minutes, until the pasta is cooked through. Garnish with parsley and serve hot.

TIP: This soup is traditionally served with warm, crusty Italian bread and cheese.

PER SERVING: *Choices/Exchanges ½ Starch, 1 Nonstarchy Vegetable, 1 Lean Protein; Calories 110 (from Fat 20); Fat 2.5g (Saturated 0.3g, Trans 0.0g); Cholesterol 0mg; Sodium 90mg; Potassium 470mg; Total Carbohydrate 16g (Dietary Fiber 4g; Sugars 4g); Protein 7g; Phosphorus 115mg.*

Lentil Soup

PREP TIME: ABOUT 10 MIN	COOK TIME: 55 MIN	SERVINGS: 8	SERVING SIZE: 1 CUP

INGREDIENTS

1 large onion, diced

1 large carrot, peeled and diced

2 stalks celery, diced

2 tablespoons extra-virgin olive oil

1 pound lentils

1½ quarts low-sodium chicken or beef broth

2 medium russet or white potatoes, peeled and diced

1 tablespoon finely chopped fresh oregano

1 teaspoon finely chopped fresh thyme

DIRECTIONS

1 In a stockpot or Dutch oven, sauté the onion, carrot, and celery in the olive oil for 10 minutes. Add the lentils, broth, and potatoes.

2 Continue to cook for 30–45 minutes, adding the oregano and thyme 15 minutes before serving. Soup will keep for 3 days in the refrigerator or can be frozen for 3 months.

TIP: Cooking with lentils is a tasty and inexpensive way to include high-quality protein and complex carbohydrates in your diet — and they're easy to use because they don't require presoaking. This is a thick, hearty soup, perfect for a chilly day.

PER SERVING: *Choices/Exchanges 2½ Starch, 1 Nonstarchy Vegetable, 1 Lean Protein; Calories 270 (from Fat 35); Fat 4g (Saturated 0.6g, Trans 0.0g); Cholesterol 0mg; Sodium 120mg; Potassium 990mg; Total Carbohydrate 41g (Dietary Fiber 14g; Sugars 5g); Protein 20g; Phosphorus 340mg.*

Mexican Tortilla Soup

PREP TIME: ABOUT 10 MIN	COOK TIME: 40 MIN	SERVINGS: 8	SERVING SIZE: 1 CUP

INGREDIENTS

2 tablespoons extra-virgin olive oil

1 onion, chopped

2 cloves garlic, minced

¼ cup freshly chopped cilantro

1 tablespoon cumin

1 teaspoon cayenne pepper

1 quart low-sodium chicken broth

One 15-ounce can low-sodium whole tomatoes, drained and coarsely chopped

1 medium zucchini, sliced

1 medium yellow squash, sliced

1 cup yellow corn

Six 6-inch corn tortillas

½ cup reduced-fat shredded cheddar cheese

DIRECTIONS

1 Preheat the oven to 350 degrees.

2 In a large saucepan, heat the oil, and sauté the onion and garlic for 5 minutes.

3 Add the cilantro, cumin, and cayenne pepper; sauté for 3 more minutes. Add the remaining ingredients except the tortillas and cheese. Bring to a boil; cover and let simmer for 30 minutes.

4 Cut each tortilla into about 10 strips (use a pizza cutter to do this easily). Place the strips on a cookie sheet and bake for 5–6 minutes at 350 degrees until slightly browned and toasted. Remove from the oven.

5 To serve the soup, place strips of tortilla into each bowl. Ladle the soup on top of the tortilla strips. Top with cheese.

PER SERVING: *Choices/Exchanges 1 Starch, 1 Nonstarchy Vegetable, 1 Fat; Calories 150 (from Fat 50); Fat 6g (Saturated 1.5g, Trans 0.0g); Cholesterol 6mg; Sodium 125mg; Potassium 420mg; Total Carbohydrate 18g (Dietary Fiber 3g; Sugars 4g); Protein 8g; Phosphorus 180mg.*

Pasta e Fagioli

PREP TIME: ABOUT 10 MIN	COOK TIME: 25 MIN	SERVINGS: 12	SERVING SIZE: 1 CUP

INGREDIENTS

1 tablespoon extra-virgin olive oil

1 large onion, chopped

3 cloves garlic, crushed

2 medium carrots, sliced

2 medium zucchini, sliced

2 tablespoons finely chopped fresh basil

2 teaspoons finely chopped fresh oregano

Two 14.5-ounce cans unsalted tomatoes with liquid

Two 15-ounce cans low-sodium white cannellini or navy beans, drained and rinsed

¾ pound whole-wheat uncooked rigatoni or shell pasta

DIRECTIONS

1 In a large saucepan, heat the oil and sauté the onion and garlic for 5 minutes.

2 Add the carrots, zucchini, basil, oregano, tomatoes with their liquid, and beans. Cook until the vegetables are just tender, about 15–17 minutes.

3 In a separate saucepan, cook the pasta according to package directions (without adding salt). Add the pasta to the soup, and mix thoroughly. Serve warm with crusty bread.

TIP: Freeze this hearty Italian soup in order to get several meals out of this recipe.

PER SERVING: *Choices/Exchanges 2 Starch, 2 Nonstarchy Vegetable; Calories 210 (from Fat 20); Fat 2g (Saturated 0.3g, Trans 0.0g); Cholesterol 0mg; Sodium 25mg; Potassium 530mg; Total Carbohydrate 40g (Dietary Fiber 8g; Sugars 6g); Protein 9g; Phosphorus 175mg.*

Manhattan Clam Chowder

| PREP TIME: ABOUT 10 MIN | COOK TIME: 1½ MIN | SERVINGS: 8 | SERVING SIZE: 1 CUP |

INGREDIENTS

3 medium carrots, peeled and coarsely chopped

3 large white or russet potatoes, peeled and coarsely chopped

4 celery stalks, coarsely chopped

2½ cups minced clams, drained

2 cups canned tomatoes, slightly crushed

½ teaspoon dried thyme or 1 teaspoon minced fresh thyme

Freshly ground black pepper

DIRECTIONS

1 Add all the ingredients to a large stockpot. Cover and let simmer for 1½ hours. Taste and add a dash of salt if needed. Serve hot.

TIP: Try serving this chunky chowder with hot sourdough bread for a great flavor and texture combo.

PER SERVING: *Choices/Exchanges 1 Starch, 1 Nonstarchy Vegetable, 1 Lean Protein; Calories 150 (from Fat 10); Fat 1g (Saturated 0.1g, Trans 0.0g); Cholesterol 35mg; Sodium 180mg; Potassium 790mg; Total Carbohydrate 21g (Dietary Fiber 3g; Sugars 4g); Protein 15g; Phosphorus 220mg.*

Quick Shrimp Gumbo

PREP TIME: ABOUT 10 MIN	COOK TIME: 40 MIN	SERVINGS: 4	SERVING SIZE: 3 OUNCES SHRIMP AND ¼ CUP RICE

INGREDIENTS

2 cups low-sodium canned tomatoes, undrained

¼ cup chopped green bell pepper

1 medium onion, chopped

1 cup cooked brown rice

½ cup low-sodium chicken broth

1 medium garlic clove, minced

Dash hot pepper sauce

Freshly ground black pepper

12 ounces precooked fresh (never frozen) jumbo shrimp

DIRECTIONS

1 Place all the ingredients except the shrimp in a large stockpot and bring to a boil. Reduce the heat, cover, and let simmer for 25–30 minutes.

2 Add the shrimp, cover, and simmer for 5–10 minutes or until the shrimp is thoroughly heated. Serve hot.

TIP: Serve this spicy gumbo with a fresh spinach salad and warm rolls.

PER SERVING: *Choices/Exchanges ½ Starch, 2 Nonstarchy Vegetable, 2 Lean Protein; Calories 190 (from Fat 10); Fat 1g (Saturated 0.2g, Trans 0.0g); Cholesterol 160mg; Sodium 125mg; Potassium 590mg; Total Carbohydrate 22g (Dietary Fiber 3g; Sugars 5g); Protein 24g; Phosphorus 295mg.*

Spanish Black Bean Soup

PREP TIME: ABOUT 5 MIN	COOK TIME: 1 HR 10 MIN	SERVINGS: 6	SERVING SIZE: 1 CUP

INGREDIENTS

1 ½ cups plus 2 teaspoons low-sodium chicken broth, divided

1 teaspoon extra-virgin olive oil

3 garlic cloves, minced

1 yellow onion, minced

1 teaspoon minced fresh oregano

1 teaspoon cumin

1 teaspoon chili powder or ½ teaspoon cayenne pepper

1 red bell pepper, chopped

1 carrot, coarsely chopped

3 cups cooked black beans

½ cup dry red wine

DIRECTIONS

1 In a large pot, heat 2 teaspoons of the chicken broth and the olive oil. Add the garlic and onion, and sauté for 3 minutes. Add the oregano, cumin, and chili powder; stir for another minute. Add the red pepper and carrot.

2 Puree 1½ cups of the black beans in a blender or food processor. Add the pureed beans, the remaining 1½ cups of whole black beans, the remaining 1½ cups of chicken broth, and the red wine to the stockpot. Simmer 1 hour.

3 Taste before serving; add additional spices if you like.

PER SERVING: *Choices/Exchanges 1½ Starch, 1 Nonstarchy Vegetable; Calories 160 (from Fat 15); Fat 1.5g (Saturated 0.3g, Trans 0.0g); Cholesterol 0mg; Sodium 55mg; Potassium 500mg; Total Carbohydrate 26g (Dietary Fiber 9g; Sugars 5g); Protein 10g; Phosphorus 160mg.*

Spicy Turkey Chili

PREP TIME: ABOUT 10 MIN | COOK TIME: 50 MIN | SERVINGS: 6 | SERVING SIZE: 1 CUP

INGREDIENTS

2 onions, chopped

2 garlic cloves, minced

½ cup chopped green bell pepper

1 tablespoon extra-virgin olive oil

1 pound lean ground turkey breast meat

2 cups cooked (not canned) kidney or pinto beans

2 cups canned tomatoes with liquid

1 cup low-sodium chicken broth

2 tablespoon chili powder

2 teaspoons cumin

Freshly ground black pepper

DIRECTIONS

1 In a large saucepan, sauté the onion, garlic, and green pepper in the oil for 10 minutes. Add the turkey, and sauté until the turkey is cooked, about 5–10 minutes. Drain any fat away.

2 Add the remaining ingredients, bring to a boil, lower the heat, and simmer uncovered for 30 minutes. Add additional chili powder if you like your chili extra spicy.

TIP: This chili tastes great with fresh-baked Corn Muffins (see Chapter 14).

PER SERVING: *Choices/Exchanges 1 Starch, 2 Nonstarchy Vegetable, 3 Lean Protein; Calories 240 (from Fat 45); Fat 5g (Saturated 0.9g, Trans 0.0g); Cholesterol 45mg; Sodium 200mg; Potassium 790mg; Total Carbohydrate 24g (Dietary Fiber 7g; Sugars 5g); Protein 27g; Phosphorus 310mg.*

White Bean Soup

PREP TIME: ABOUT 5 MIN | COOK TIME: 2½ HR | SERVINGS: 6 | SERVING SIZE: 1 CUP

INGREDIENTS

¼ cup chopped onion

1 garlic clove, minced

2 tablespoons extra-virgin olive oil

½ pound dried great northern, white navy, or cannellini beans, soaked in boiling water for 1 hour and drained

2 quarts water

2 bay leaves

1 teaspoon dried basil

1/16 teaspoon salt

1/16 teaspoon freshly ground black pepper

2 medium scallions, chopped

2 tablespoons minced fresh parsley

DIRECTIONS

1 In a large saucepan, sauté the onion and garlic in the oil for 5 minutes. Add the beans, water, bay leaves, and basil; stir well. Bring the mixture to a boil, reduce the heat, cover, and let simmer.

2 Continue to cook the soup for 1–1½ hours or until the beans are tender. Add water (if necessary), salt, and pepper; mix well.

3 Remove and discard the bay leaves. In a blender or food processor, puree the mixture. Return the soup to the saucepan and serve hot. Garnish with scallions and parsley.

VARY IT! Use any variety of white bean for this scrumptious soup.

PER SERVING: *Choices/Exchanges 1½ Starch, 1 Lean Protein; Calories 150 (from Fat 45); Fat 5g (Saturated 0.8g, Trans 0.0g); Cholesterol 0mg; Sodium 25mg; Potassium 390mg; Total Carbohydrate 20g (Dietary Fiber 7g; Sugars 2g); Protein 8g; Phosphorous 155mg.*

Chapter **6**

Pasta

RECIPES IN THIS CHAPTER

I f you think having diabetes means eliminating pasta from your diet, think again! Pasta dishes are a family favorite. They're rich, filling, fun to eat, and often easy to prepare. But pasta has a reputation for being unhealthy.

Traditional pasta dishes *are* high in carbohydrate and often contain high-fat ingredients, but you don't have to take pasta off the table completely. The recipes in this chapter are great, healthier alternatives to heavy pasta dishes.

Making a few simple changes to your average pasta dish can transform it into a balanced and nutritious meal. For example, using whole-wheat pasta instead of regular pasta can increase the dish's fiber content, and adding nonstarchy vegetables to a recipe is a great way to make it hearty and flavorful without a lot of extra carbohydrate. The recipes in this chapter take advantage of these and other healthy changes to bring you diabetes-friendly pasta dishes that everyone will love!

REMEMBER

People with diabetes can still eat all kinds of foods. The key is moderation! So, if you're craving a favorite dish or a rich dessert, it's okay to indulge once in a while. Just make sure you control your portion sizes and account for the dish in your diabetes meal plan. It's probably best to save these treats for special occasions, but it's important to enjoy the foods you love.

Fusilli with Sage and Peppers

PREP TIME: ABOUT 10 MIN	COOK TIME: 20 MIN	SERVINGS: 8	SERVING SIZE: 1 CUP

INGREDIENTS

2 tablespoons chicken broth

1 garlic clove, minced

½ cup chopped onion

½ red bell pepper, cut into thin strips

½ green bell pepper, cut into thin strips

½ yellow bell pepper, cut into thin strips

2 tablespoons chopped fresh sage

One 15-ounce can tomato puree

1 tablespoon tomato paste

2 tablespoons red wine

1 teaspoon crushed red pepper (optional)

1 pound cooked (al dente) whole-wheat fusilli

DIRECTIONS

1 In a large skillet over medium heat, heat the broth. Add the garlic and onion, and sauté for 5–8 minutes. Add the peppers, and sauté for another 7 minutes.

2 Add the sage, tomato puree, tomato paste, red wine, and red pepper. Lower the heat to a simmer, and cook for 15 minutes.

3 Add the cooked pasta, and let stand for 5 minutes. Serve.

VARY IT! Quinoa pasta and cooked barley would make great alternatives to the whole-wheat fusilli in this recipe. Other garden vegetables, like zucchini and eggplant, would also work well in this sauce.

PER SERVING: *Choices/Exchanges 1 Starch, 2 Nonstarchy Vegetable; Calories 120 (from Fat 5); Fat 0.5g (Saturated 0.1g, Trans 0.0g); Cholesterol 0 mg; Sodium 50mg; Potassium 360mg, Total Carbohydrate 24g (Dietary Fiber 4g; Sugars 5g); Protein 5g; Phosphorus 85mg.*

Eggplant Lasagna

PREP TIME: ABOUT 15 MIN	COOK TIME: 1 HR 20 MIN	SERVINGS: 6	SERVING SIZE: 1 (4½-INCH) SQUARE

INGREDIENTS

1 tablespoon extra-virgin olive oil, divided

1¾ cups chopped onion

2 medium garlic cloves, minced

One 14.5-ounce can no-salt-added diced tomatoes, undrained

5 tablespoons no-salt-added tomato paste

½ cup water

2 tablespoons freshly chopped parsley

1 teaspoon finely chopped fresh oregano

4 tablespoons finely chopped fresh basil

Freshly ground black pepper

1 large (1½-pound) eggplant, peeled and sliced into ¼-inch slices

1 cup shredded reduced-fat mozzarella cheese

1 cup nonfat ricotta

4 tablespoons freshly grated Parmigiano-Reggiano cheese

DIRECTIONS

1 Preheat the oven to 350 degrees.

2 Coat a large skillet with ½ tablespoon of the olive oil. Add the onion and garlic, and sauté over low heat until the onion is tender, about 6 minutes.

3 Stir in the tomatoes, tomato paste, water, parsley, oregano, basil, and pepper. Bring the mixture to a boil. Reduce the heat and simmer, covered, for 30 minutes, stirring occasionally.

4 To steam the eggplant slices, place 1 inch of water in a large pot. Arrange the eggplant slices on a steamer, cover the pot, and steam until the eggplant is tender, about 5 minutes. Do not overcook.

5 In a medium bowl, combine the mozzarella and ricotta cheese together, and set aside.

6 Coat a 13-x-9-x-2-inch baking pan with the remaining ½ tablespoon olive oil, and place half of the eggplant in the pan. Top the eggplant with half of the cheese mixture and half of the sauce, and sprinkle with half of the Parmigiano-Reggiano cheese. Repeat.

7 Bake at 350 degrees for 30–35 minutes, and serve hot.

TIP: This hearty vegetarian entree can be made ahead and frozen.

PER SERVING: *Choices/Exchanges 4 Nonstarchy Vegetable, 1 Lean Protein, 1 Fat; Calories 180 (from Fat 60); Fat 7g (Saturated 3.1g, Trans 0.0g); Cholesterol 25mg; Sodium 220mg; Potassium 530mg; Total Carbohydrate 20g (Dietary Fiber 4g; Sugars 10g); Protein 14g; Phosphorus 240mg.*

Fettuccine with Peppers and Broccoli

| PREP TIME: ABOUT 5 MIN | COOK TIME: 20 MIN | SERVINGS: 4 | SERVING SIZE: 1 CUP |

INGREDIENTS

2 tablespoons extra-virgin olive oil

2 medium garlic cloves, minced

2 large red bell peppers, halved, seeded, and cut into ½-inch strips

6 ounces whole-wheat fettuccine

1¾ pounds fresh broccoli florets, washed

¼ cup Parmigiano-Reggiano cheese

DIRECTIONS

1 In a large skillet over medium heat, heat the olive oil. Add the garlic, and sauté for 1 minute. Add the peppers and continue sautéing for 3–5 minutes or until the peppers are just tender, stirring occasionally. Remove from the heat, and set aside.

2 Prepare the fettucine according to package directions (without adding salt) and drain.

3 Add the broccoli to a large pot of boiling water, and then turn off the heat. After 1 minute, rinse the broccoli under cold running water to stop the cooking process; drain. (This method of blanching helps the broccoli to retain its bright green color and crispness.)

4 In a large bowl, toss the fettucine with the peppers, and arrange the broccoli on top. Sprinkle with the Parmigiano-Reggiano cheese, and serve.

PER SERVING: *Choices/Exchanges 2 Starch, 3 Nonstarchy Vegetable, 1 Lean Protein; Calories 320 (from Fat 90); Fat 10g (Saturated 2.2g, Trans 0.0g); Cholesterol 10mg; Sodium 95mg; Potassium 940mg; Total Carbohydrate 47g (Dietary Fiber 12g; Sugars 9g); Protein 15g, Phosphorus 300mg.*

Garlic Fettuccine

PREP TIME: ABOUT 5 MIN | **COOK TIME: 30 MIN** | **SERVINGS: 5** | **SERVING SIZE: 1 CUP**

INGREDIENTS

2 tablespoons extra-virgin olive oil

12 plum tomatoes, seeded and diced

4 cloves garlic, minced

¼ teaspoon salt

Freshly ground black pepper

1 teaspoon capers

2 teaspoons pitted black olives (such as Kalamata), chopped

6 ounces whole-wheat fettuccine (made without egg)

¼ cup chopped fresh basil

Freshly chopped parsley, for garnish

DIRECTIONS

1 In a large saucepan over medium heat, heat the oil. Add the tomatoes, garlic, salt, pepper, capers, and olives. Let simmer over low heat for 30 minutes, stirring occasionally.

2 Prepare the fettuccine according to package directions (without adding salt) and drain. Transfer the fettucine to a serving bowl and spoon the sauce and chopped basil on top. Garnish with parsley to serve.

PER SERVING: *Choices/Exchanges 1½ Starch, 1 Nonstarchy Vegetable, 1½ Fat; Calories 210 (from Fat 60); Fat 7g (Saturated 0.9g, Trans 0.0g); Cholesterol 0mg; Sodium 160mg; Potassium 410mg; Total Carbohydrate 31g (Dietary Fiber 5g; Sugars 4g); Protein 7g, Phosphorus 125mg.*

Pasta with Vegetable Clam Sauce

PREP TIME: ABOUT 5 MIN	COOK TIME: 10 MIN	SERVINGS: 8	SERVING SIZE: ½ CUP PASTA PLUS 2 TABLESPOONS SAUCE

INGREDIENTS

2 tablespoons extra-virgin olive oil

5 medium cloves garlic, crushed

4 celery stalks, chopped

2 small zucchini, thinly sliced

4 scallions, chopped

¼ pound fresh mushrooms, sliced

2 tablespoons chopped fresh parsley

One 7-ounce can clams, undrained

2 small tomatoes, chopped

⅓ cup dry white wine

2 tablespoons fresh lemon juice

Freshly ground black pepper

1 pound cooked whole-wheat rigatoni or shells

DIRECTIONS

1 In a large skillet over medium heat, heat the oil. Sauté the garlic until lightly browned. Add the celery, zucchini, scallions, mushrooms, and parsley; sauté until the vegetables are just tender (about 5 minutes).

2 Add the clams with their juice, tomatoes, wine, lemon juice, and pepper; stir well. Let simmer, uncovered, for 4–5 minutes.

3 Place the cooked pasta on a serving platter. Remove the sauce from the heat and spoon over the pasta. Sprinkle with a dash of Parmigiano–Reggiano cheese (optional), and serve.

TIP: Cook pasta to al dente for better texture and nutrition.

PER SERVING: *Choices/Exchanges 1½ Starch, 1 Nonstarchy Vegetable, 1 Fat; Calories 180 (from Fat 40); Fat 4.5g (Saturated 0.6g, Trans 0.0g); Cholesterol 10mg; Sodium 75mg; Potassium 410mg; Total Carbohydrate 28g (Dietary Fiber 4g; Sugars 3g); Protein 8g; Phosphorus 145mg.*

Rigatoni with Chicken and Vegetables

PREP TIME: ABOUT 15 MIN	COOK TIME: 15 MIN	SERVINGS: 8	SERVING SIZE: 1 PIECE CHICKEN AND ¾ CUP PASTA WITH SAUCE

INGREDIENTS

12 ounces whole-wheat rigatoni (or substitute any other shaped pasta)

¼ cup extra-virgin olive oil

1 medium onion, chopped

1 large green bell pepper, julienned

1 large red bell pepper, julienned

1 large yellow bell pepper, julienned

2 garlic cloves, minced

2 tomatoes, chopped

½ cup low-sodium chicken broth

¼ cup minced fresh parsley

2 tablespoons finely chopped fresh basil

Dash crushed red pepper

2 tablespoons lemon juice

2 pounds boneless, skinless chicken breasts, cut into about 8 pieces, and cooked

DIRECTIONS

1 Cook the rigatoni according to package directions (without adding salt), drain, and set aside.

2 In a large skillet over medium heat, heat the oil. Add the onion, peppers, and garlic, and sauté for 6 minutes.

3 Add the tomatoes, chicken broth, parsley, basil, crushed red pepper, and salt and pepper if desired. Add the lemon juice. Add the chicken to the skillet, and cook the chicken in the sauce over low heat just until the chicken is warmed in the sauce.

4 Arrange the cooked rigatoni on a serving platter. Spoon the chicken and pepper sauce over the rigatoni and serve.

PER SERVING: *Choices/Exchanges 2 Starch, 2 Nonstarchy Vegetable, 3 Lean Protein, 1 Fat; Calories 380 (from Fat 100); Fat 11g (Saturated 1.9g, Trans 0.0g); Cholesterol 65mg; Sodium 80mg; Potassium 570mg; Total Carbohydrate 41g (Dietary Fiber 7g; Sugars 6g); Protein 31g, Phosphorus 320mg.*

Spaghetti and Artichoke Pie

PREP TIME: ABOUT 5 MIN	COOK TIME: 20 MIN	SERVINGS: 4	SERVING SIZE: 1 WEDGE

INGREDIENTS

3 cups cooked whole-wheat spaghetti

1 cup frozen artichokes, drained

2 egg whites

2 tablespoons fat-free milk

¼ cup freshly grated Parmigiano-Reggiano cheese

1 teaspoon freshly chopped oregano

2 teaspoons freshly chopped basil

2 teaspoons freshly chopped mint

DIRECTIONS

1 Preheat the oven to 350 degrees.

2 In a medium bowl, combine all the ingredients, and mix well.

3 Pour the spaghetti mixture into an ovenproof nonstick round casserole dish or skillet, and spread evenly.

4 Bake the pie, uncovered, at 350 degrees until golden brown, about 20 minutes. Cut into 4 wedges, and serve.

TIP: This is a great way to use leftover spaghetti.

PER SERVING: *Choices/Exchanges 2 Starch, 1 Nonstarchy Vegetable; Calories 180 (from Fat 20); Fat 2.0g (Saturated 1.2g, Trans 0.0g); Cholesterol 2mg; Sodium 85mg; Potassium 200mg, Total Carbohydrate 32g (Dietary Fiber 6g; Sugars 2g); Protein 10g, Phosphorus 165mg.*

Linguine with Pesto Sauce

PREP TIME: ABOUT 5 MIN | **SERVINGS: 6** | **SERVING SIZE: ½ CUP**

INGREDIENTS

3 cups fresh basil, stems removed

3 garlic cloves, chopped

¼ cup extra-virgin olive oil

1 cup pine nuts, toasted

¼ cup Parmigiano-Reggiano cheese

Freshly ground black pepper

1 pound cooked whole-wheat linguine, hot

DIRECTIONS

1 Wash and dry the basil. Place the basil in a blender or food processor with the garlic, olive oil, pine nuts, cheese, and pepper, and process until smooth.

2 Transfer the cooked linguine to a serving bowl. Add the pesto, and toss thoroughly to serve.

VARY IT! Swap fresh basil for spinach and pine nuts for almonds to vary this delicious recipe.

TIP: Pesto sauce should never be heated. In addition to pasta, it is a great topping for vegetables, fish, and chicken.

PER SERVING: *Choices/Exchanges ½ Starch, 2 Fat; Calories 130 (from Fat 90); Fat 10g (Saturated 1.2g, Trans 0.0g); Cholesterol 0mg; Sodium 10mg; Potassium 105mg; Total Carbohydrate 9g (Dietary Fiber 2g; Sugars 1g); Protein 3g; Phosphorus 90mg.*

Stuffed Manicotti

PREP TIME: ABOUT 10 MIN	COOK TIME: 20 MIN	SERVINGS: 4	SERVING SIZE: 2 STUFFED MANICOTTI SHELLS

INGREDIENTS

2 tablespoons low-sodium chicken broth

½ cup minced onion

½ cup minced carrot

1 cup minced celery

1 garlic clove, minced

1 cup low-fat ricotta cheese

¼ cup egg substitute

2 tablespoons Parmigiano-Reggiano cheese

1 tablespoon chopped fresh basil

8 large whole-wheat manicotti shells, cooked

2 cups Marinara Sauce (see recipe later in this chapter)

DIRECTIONS

1 Preheat the oven to 350 degrees.

2 In a skillet over medium heat, heat the broth. Add the onion, carrot, celery, and garlic, and sauté for 5–7 minutes, until the onion is tender.

3 In a large bowl, combine the vegetables with the ricotta cheese, egg substitute, Parmigiano–Reggiano cheese, and basil. Mix well.

4 Stuff some of the mixture into each shell. Place the stuffed manicotti shells in a large casserole dish. Pour the marinara sauce on top, and let cook at 350 degrees for 20 minutes.

VARY IT! You can also use the filling in this recipe for lasagna or stuffed shells.

PER SERVING: *Choices/Exchanges 2 Starch, 1 Nonstarchy Vegetable, 1 Lean Protein, ½ Fat; Calories 250 (from Fat 35); Fat 4g (Saturated 2.2g, Trans 0.0g); Cholesterol 20mg; Sodium 200mg; Potassium 690mg; Total Carbohydrate 40g (Dietary Fiber 7g; Sugars 10g); Protein 16g, Phosphorus 285mg.*

Vegetable Lo Mein

PREP TIME: ABOUT 15 MIN	COOK TIME: 10 MIN	SERVINGS: 8	SERVING SIZE: 1 CUP

INGREDIENTS

1 cup plus 2 tablespoons low-sodium chicken broth

2 garlic cloves, minced

¼ cup minced scallions

2 teaspoons grated fresh ginger

2 carrots, peeled and cut into ¼-inch slices

3 celery stalks, cut on the diagonal into ¼-inch slices

½ cup sliced mushrooms

1½ cups broccoli florets

2 tablespoons dry sherry

1 tablespoon light soy sauce

1 teaspoon sesame oil

1 tablespoon cornstarch

½ pound cooked whole-wheat vermicelli

DIRECTIONS

1 In a large skillet or wok, heat 2 tablespoons of the broth. Add the garlic, scallions, and ginger, and sauté for 30 seconds.

2 Add the carrots, celery, and mushrooms, and sauté for 5 minutes. Add the broccoli and ½ cup of the broth, cover, and steam for 5 minutes.

3 In a small bowl, combine the remaining ½ cup of broth with the sherry, soy sauce, and sesame oil. Add the cornstarch, and mix well.

4 Remove the cover, and add the cornstarch mixture. Cook for 1 minute more until the mixture thickens. Toss in the cooked noodles, and mix well. Serve.

VARY IT! Swap out vermicelli for rice for a delicious Asian stir-fry.

PER SERVING: *Choices/Exchanges ½ Starch, 1 Nonstarchy Vegetable; Calories 80 (from Fat 10); Fat 1g (Saturated 0.2g, Trans 0.0g); Cholesterol 0mg; Sodium 120mg; Potassium 240mg; Total Carbohydrate 13g (Dietary Fiber 2g; Sugars 2g); Protein 4g; Phosphorus 75mg.*

Marinara Sauce

PREP TIME: ABOUT 5 MIN	COOK TIME: 40–50 MIN	SERVINGS: 20	SERVING SIZE: ¼ CUP

INGREDIENTS

One 28-ounce can no-salt-added crushed tomatoes

1 green bell pepper, chopped

1 red bell pepper, chopped

½ cup minced onion

1 teaspoon dried oregano

½ pound mushrooms, sliced

1 teaspoon dried basil

½ teaspoon garlic powder

DIRECTIONS

1 In a large saucepan over medium heat, combine all the ingredients, mixing thoroughly.

2 Let simmer 40–50 minutes, allowing flavors to blend.

TIP: Keep a batch of this sauce on hand in the freezer. The taste complements shrimp or pasta and is a great dipping sauce for baked chicken fingers.

PER SERVING: *Choices/Exchanges 1 Nonstarchy Vegetable; Calories 25 (from Fat 0); Fat 0g (Saturated 0.0g, Trans 0.0g); Cholesterol 0mg; Sodium 5mg; Potassium 200mg; Total Carbohydrate 5g (Dietary Fiber 2g; Sugars 2g); Protein 1g, Phosphorus 30mg.*

Chapter **7**

Poultry

Lean cuts of poultry make quick, delicious meals and are a great protein option for people with diabetes. From fun and tasty chicken tenders to juicy turkey burgers, nothing says "family favorite" like poultry. The healthiest poultry choices for people with diabetes are white meat cuts like breasts and tenderloins with the skin removed. Dark meat cuts and duck contain more fat, so it's a good idea to enjoy these in moderation.

The recipes in this chapter were designed to showcase the flavors of chicken, turkey, and even Cornish hens without compromising your healthy eating efforts. They incorporate lean cuts of poultry with healthy cooking methods — you won't find greasy fried chicken in this chapter — and both classic and more exotic flavor profiles to create dishes you'll love to cook again and again.

Mediterranean-Style Chicken Scaloppine

PREP TIME: ABOUT 15 MIN PLUS MARINATING TIME	COOK TIME: 1 HR	SERVINGS: 6	SERVING SIZE: 3 OUNCES

INGREDIENTS

Six 3-ounce boneless, skinless chicken breast halves

2 cups fat-free Greek yogurt

¼ cup lemon juice

Zest of 1 lemon

¼ cup freshly chopped baby dill

2 teaspoons paprika

2 garlic cloves, minced

$\frac{1}{16}$ teaspoon salt

¼ teaspoon freshly ground black pepper

1 cup dried whole-wheat bread crumbs

2½ cups frozen artichoke hearts, thawed

2 tablespoons extra-virgin olive oil

¼ cup finely chopped fresh parsley

1 lemon, sliced

DIRECTIONS

1 Wash chicken breasts under cold running water, and pat dry.

2 In a medium bowl, combine the yogurt, lemon juice, lemon zest, baby dill, paprika, garlic, salt, and pepper. Measure out ½ cup of this marinade, and reserve the rest in the refrigerator.

3 Add the chicken to the ½ cup of marinade, and coat each piece well. Refrigerate overnight.

4 Preheat the oven to 350 degrees.

5 Remove the chicken from the marinade, discard the marinade, and roll the chicken in bread crumbs, coating evenly.

6 Arrange the chicken in a single layer in a large baking pan. Add the artichoke hearts in with the chicken. Drizzle the olive oil over the chicken and artichokes. Bake at 350 degrees, uncovered, for 45 minutes, or until the chicken is no longer pink.

7 Transfer to a serving platter, and serve with the remaining marinade as a sauce and parsley and lemon slices as a garnish.

VARY IT! Turkey breast and cod filets also work well with this recipe.

PER SERVING: *Choices/Exchanges 1 Starch, 1 Nonstarchy Vegetable, 3 Lean Protein, ½ Fat; Calories 260 (from Fat 70); Fat 8g (Saturated 1.4g, Trans 0.0g); Cholesterol 50mg; Sodium 140mg; Potassium 500mg; Total Carbohydrate 21g (Dietary Fiber 5g, Sugars 4g); Protein 29g; Phosphorus 295mg.*

Roasted Chicken Kiev

PREP TIME: 30 MIN PLUS 4 HR FREEZING TIME	COOK TIME: 45 MIN	SERVINGS: 6	SERVING SIZE: 3 OUNCES

INGREDIENTS

¼ cup extra-virgin olive oil

¼ cup freshly chopped parsley

½ teaspoon dried rosemary

4 cloves garlic, minced

¹⁄₁₆ teaspoon salt

¼ teaspoon freshly ground black pepper

Three 8-ounce boneless, skinless chicken breasts, halved

¼ cup fat-free milk

⅓ cup dried bread crumbs

1 lemon, cut into wedges

DIRECTIONS

1 With a whisk, combine the olive oil, parsley, rosemary, garlic, salt, and pepper in a small mixing bowl. Divide the mixture evenly into 6 ice cube tray compartments; freeze until firm (approximately 4 hours).

2 Preheat the oven to 400 degrees. Place each chicken breast half between 2 sheets of wax paper and flatten to ¼-inch thickness with a meat mallet or rolling pin.

3 Place an oil cube in the center of each chicken breast; fold the ends over the oil and roll up, beginning with the long side. Secure each end with wooden toothpicks.

4 Dip the chicken rolls into the milk and coat thoroughly with bread crumbs. Transfer to a 9-x-13-inch baking dish. Bake at 400 degrees for 25 minutes until browned.

5 Arrange the chicken on a serving platter, spoon the juices from the pan over the top, garnish with the lemon wedges, and serve.

TIP: This low-fat version of a classic dish is great to serve when entertaining.

PER SERVING: *Choices/Exchanges ½ Starch, 3 Lean Protein, 1½ Fat; Calories 240 (from Fat 110); Fat 12g (Saturated 2.1g, Trans 0.0g); Cholesterol 65mg; Sodium 130mg; Potassium 250mg; Total Carbohydrate 6g (Dietary Fiber 0g, Sugars 1g); Protein 25g; Phosphorus 200mg.*

Baked Chicken with Wine Sauce

PREP TIME: ABOUT 5 MIN	COOK TIME: 1 HR 20 MIN	SERVINGS: 8	SERVING SIZE: ONE 3- TO 4-OUNCE PIECE CHICKEN PLUS SAUCE

INGREDIENTS

2 tablespoons extra-virgin olive oil, divided

Four 8-ounce boneless, skinless chicken breasts, halved

2 tablespoons flour

½ cup low-sodium chicken broth

¾ cup plain fat-free Greek yogurt

¼ cup dry white wine

Zest of 1 lemon

¼ teaspoon salt

¼ teaspoon freshly ground black pepper

1 teaspoon minced fresh thyme

½ teaspoon ground sage

½ cup sliced mushrooms

4 tablespoons finely chopped fresh parsley sprigs

DIRECTIONS

1 Preheat the oven to 350 degrees. Grease a shallow baking dish with 1 tablespoon of olive oil; place the chicken breasts in the dish. Bake uncovered for 30 minutes.

2 Meanwhile, heat the remaining olive oil in a medium sauce-pan over medium heat. Add the flour, and stir until smooth. Add the chicken broth, and stir until the mixture is thickened. Add the yogurt, wine, lemon zest, salt, pepper, thyme, and sage. Stir until completely smooth.

3 Remove the chicken from the oven, and turn the chicken breasts over. Cover the chicken with the mushrooms, and pour the sauce over the top. Continue to bake, uncovered, for another 30 minutes or until the chicken is no longer pink. Transfer the chicken to a serving platter, spoon the sauce over the chicken, garnish with parsley sprigs, and serve.

VARY IT! This wine sauce is also delicious with turkey or Cornish game hens.

PER SERVING: *Choices/Exchanges 4 Lean Protein; Calories 180 (from Fat 50); Fat 6g (Saturated 1.3g, Trans 0.0g); Cholesterol 65mg; Sodium 150mg; Potassium 270mg; Total Carbohydrate 3g (Dietary Fiber 0g, Sugars 1g); Protein 27g; Phosphorus 215mg.*

Chicken and Vegetable Stir-Fry

PREP TIME: ABOUT 10 MIN	COOK TIME: 20 MIN	SERVINGS: 8	SERVING SIZE: ONE 3- TO 4-OUNCE CHICKEN BREAST PLUS ½ CUP VEGETABLES/SAUCE

INGREDIENTS

1 tablespoon extra-virgin olive oil

Four 8-ounce boneless, skinless chicken breasts, cut into thin strips about ⅛ inch wide

2 garlic cloves, minced

2 teaspoons grated fresh ginger

1 tablespoon light soy sauce

1 cup sliced celery

1 cup sliced fresh mushrooms

2 cup julienned zucchini

2 teaspoons cornstarch

DIRECTIONS

1 In a large skillet or wok, heat the oil. Add the chicken, garlic, and ginger. Stir-fry until the chicken turns white, about 5 minutes.

2 Stir in the soy sauce, celery, mushrooms, and zucchini. Cover, and continue to cook for about 5 minutes.

3 In a small bowl, mix the cornstarch and 3 tablespoons of water until well combined. Slowly add this mixture to the chicken, stirring constantly. Continue to cook for 2–5 minutes, until mixture is thickened. Remove from the heat, and serve.

VARY IT! You can also use squash and red or green bell peppers in the recipe. It works well with turkey breast, too.

PER SERVING: *Choices/Exchanges 3 Lean Protein; Calories 160 (from Fat 40); Fat 4.5g (Saturated 1.0g, Trans 0.0g); Cholesterol 65mg; Sodium 140mg; Potassium 340mg; Total Carbohydrate 3g (Dietary Fiber 1g, Sugars 1g); Protein 25g; Phosphorus 200mg.*

Chicken Paprika

PREP TIME: ABOUT 5 MIN	COOK TIME: 35 MIN	SERVINGS: 8	SERVING SIZE: ONE 3- TO 4-OUNCE PIECE CHICKEN PLUS SAUCE

INGREDIENTS

1 tablespoon extra-virgin olive oil

1 large onion, minced

1 medium red bell pepper, julienned

1 cup sliced fresh mushrooms

1–2 teaspoons smoked paprika

2 tablespoons lemon juice

$\frac{1}{16}$ teaspoon salt

$\frac{1}{8}$ teaspoon freshly ground black pepper

Four 8-ounce boneless, skinless chicken breasts, halved

8 ounces plain low-fat Greek yogurt

DIRECTIONS

1 Heat the oil in a large skillet over medium heat. Add the onion, red pepper, and mushrooms, and sauté until tender, about 3–4 minutes.

2 Add 1 cup of water, the paprika, lemon juice, salt, and pepper, blending well. Bring the mixture to a boil over high heat, and reduce the heat to medium. Add the chicken; cover, and let simmer for 25–30 minutes or until the chicken is no longer pink.

3 Reduce the heat to low, quickly stir in the Greek yogurt, mixing well, and continue to cook for 1–2 minutes. Do not boil. Serve hot.

TIP: It is important not to let the Greek yogurt boil or it will curdle. This healthful rendition of a Hungarian classic tastes great served with rice, barley, or other whole grains.

PER SERVING: *Choices/Exchanges 1 Nonstarchy Vegetable, 4 Lean Protein; Calories 180 (from Fat 45); Fat 5g (Saturated 1.4g, Trans 0.0g); Cholesterol 65mg; Sodium 90mg; Potassium 350mg; Total Carbohydrate 6g (Dietary Fiber 1g, Sugars 3g); Protein 27g; Phosphorus 235mg.*

Chicken Parmesan

PREP TIME: ABOUT 5 MIN	COOK TIME: 45 MIN	SERVINGS: 6	SERVING SIZE: ONE 3-OUNCE PIECE CHICKEN PLUS SAUCE

INGREDIENTS

Six 3-ounce boneless, skinless chicken breast halves

½ cup plain soft bread crumbs

2 tablespoons freshly grated Parmigiano-Reggiano cheese

¼ teaspoon freshly ground black pepper

1 egg beaten with ¼ cup water in a shallow bowl

2 tablespoons extra-virgin olive oil

1½ cups Marinara Sauce (see Chapter 6)

1 cup shredded skim-milk mozzarella

DIRECTIONS

1 Preheat the oven to 425 degrees. Place the chicken breasts on a cutting board, and pound with a meat hammer until thin.

2 In a shallow dish, combine the bread crumbs, Parmesan cheese, and pepper.

3 Dip the chicken breasts into the egg mixture and then the crumb mixture, coating both sides.

4 In a large nonstick skillet, heat the oil. Add the chicken, and sauté until golden brown, about 4–5 minutes on each side or until the chicken is no longer pink. Transfer the chicken to a shallow baking pan.

5 Pour the sauce over the chicken, and sprinkle mozzarella over the top.

6 Bake at 425 degrees for 20–25 minutes or until mozzarella is melted and slightly golden.

TIP: This dish tastes great with Garlic Fettuccine (see Chapter 6) and Fettuccine with Peppers and Broccoli (see Chapter 6).

PER SERVING: *Choices/Exchanges 1 Nonstarchy Vegetable, 3 Lean Protein, 1½ Fat; Calories 230 (from Fat 100); Fat 11g (Saturated 3.7g, Trans 0.0g); Cholesterol 95mg; Sodium 210mg; Potassium 380mg; Total Carbohydrate 7g (Dietary Fiber 2g, Sugars 3g); Protein 25g; Phosphorus 275mg.*

Chicken Provençal

PREP TIME: ABOUT 5 MIN	COOK TIME: 25 MIN	SERVINGS: 4	SERVING SIZE: 3–4 OUNCES

INGREDIENTS

2 tablespoons extra-virgin olive oil

Two 8-ounce boneless, skinless chicken breasts, halved

1 medium garlic clove, minced

¼ cup minced onion

¼ cup minced green bell pepper

½ cup dry white wine

1 cup canned diced tomatoes

¼ cup pitted Kalamata olives

¼ cup finely chopped fresh basil

⅛ teaspoon freshly ground black pepper

DIRECTIONS

1 Heat the oil in a skillet over medium heat. Add the chicken, and brown about 3–5 minutes.

2 Add the remaining ingredients, and cook uncovered over medium heat for 20 minutes or until the chicken is no longer pink. Transfer to a serving platter and season with additional pepper to taste, if desired, before serving.

VARY IT! Fish filets and vegetables such as zucchini and eggplant also work well in this recipe.

PER SERVING: *Choices/Exchanges 1 Nonstarchy Vegetable, 3 Lean Protein, 1½ Fat; Calories 240 (from Fat 110); Fat 12g (Saturated 2.0g, Trans 0.0g); Cholesterol 65mg; Sodium 280mg; Potassium 380mg; Total Carbohydrate 5g (Dietary Fiber 1g, Sugars 3g); Protein 24g; Phosphorus 195mg.*

Lemon Chicken

PREP TIME: ABOUT 5 MIN	COOK TIME: 35 MIN	SERVINGS: 6	SERVING SIZE: 3–4 OUNCES

INGREDIENTS

Three 8-ounce boneless, skinless chicken breasts, halved

1 cup dried bread crumbs

Nonstick cooking spray

¼ cup extra-virgin olive oil

¼ cup low-sodium chicken broth

Grated zest of 1 lemon

3 medium garlic cloves, minced

½ cup fresh lemon juice

½ cup water

¼ cup minced fresh oregano

1 medium lemon, cut into wedges

¼ cup minced fresh parsley, divided

DIRECTIONS

1 Preheat the oven to 325 degrees. Rinse the chicken in cold water, and then roll it in the bread crumbs.

2 Spray a skillet with nonstick cooking spray, and brown the coated chicken breasts over medium heat about 3 minutes on each side. Transfer the browned chicken to a baking dish.

3 In a small bowl, combine the remaining ingredients, except the lemon and parsley. Pour the sauce over the chicken. Bake the chicken at 325 degrees, uncovered, for 30 minutes until the chicken is no longer pink.

4 Transfer to a serving platter, and spoon the sauce over the chicken. Garnish with the lemon and parsley.

TIP: Try serving this dish with orzo (a rice-shaped pasta) and good, crusty French bread.

PER SERVING: *Choices/Exchanges 1 Starch, 3 Lean Protein, 1½ Fat; Calories 280 (from Fat 120); Fat 13g (Saturated 2.2g, Trans 0.0g); Cholesterol 65mg; Sodium 190mg; Potassium 290mg; Total Carbohydrate 14g (Dietary Fiber 1g, Sugars 2g); Protein 26g; Phosphorus 210mg.*

Chicken with Mushroom Cream Sauce

PREP TIME: ABOUT 5 MIN	COOK TIME: 20 MIN	SERVINGS: 8	SERVING SIZE: 3 OUNCES

INGREDIENTS

1 tablespoon extra-virgin olive oil

Eight 3-ounce boneless, skinless chicken breast halves

½ cup sliced mushrooms

3 tablespoons flour

½ cup low-sodium chicken broth

¾ cup white wine

2 teaspoons lemon zest

½ teaspoons lemon pepper

1 cup plain fat-free Greek yogurt

Parsley sprigs

DIRECTIONS

1 In a large nonstick skillet, heat the oil; add the chicken and cook for 5 minutes on each side. Remove the chicken, and keep warm. Add the mushrooms to the skillet, and cook until tender.

2 In a small bowl, whisk the flour with the broth and wine. Stir the mixture into the skillet, and add the lemon zest and pepper. Cook until thickened and bubbly.

3 Return the chicken to the skillet, and cook until the chicken is no longer pink. Transfer the chicken to a platter. Stir the yogurt into the skillet and heat thoroughly. Pour the sauce over the chicken, and garnish with parsley.

TIP: This dish is good with green beans, asparagus, and broccoli sautéed in olive oil.

PER SERVING: *Choices/Exchanges 3 Lean Protein; Calories 150 (from Fat 35); Fat 4g (Saturated 0.8g, Trans 0.0g); Cholesterol 50mg; Sodium 85mg; Potassium 220mg; Total Carbohydrate 4g (Dietary Fiber 0g, Sugars 1g); Protein 21g; Phosphorus 180mg.*

Grilled Herb Chicken with Wine and Roasted Garlic

PREP TIME: ABOUT 5 MIN PLUS MARINATING TIME	COOK TIME: 45 MIN	SERVINGS: 4	SERVING SIZE: 3 OUNCES

INGREDIENTS

Four 3-ounce boneless, skinless chicken breast halves

2 tablespoons extra-virgin olive oil, divided

1 cup red wine

3 sprigs fresh thyme

5 garlic cloves, minced

5 garlic cloves, whole and unpeeled

⅛ teaspoon freshly ground black pepper

DIRECTIONS

1 In a plastic zippered bag, place chicken, 1 tablespoon of the oil, wine, thyme, and minced garlic. Marinate for 2–3 hours in the refrigerator.

2 Preheat the oven to 375 degrees.

3 Spread the whole garlic cloves on a cookie sheet, drizzle with the remaining oil, and sprinkle with pepper. Bake for 30 minutes, stirring occasionally, until soft.

4 When cool, squeeze the garlic paste from the cloves, and mash in a small bowl with a fork.

5 Remove the chicken from the marinade, and grill for 12–15 minutes, turning frequently and brushing with garlic paste. Transfer to a platter, and serve hot.

PER SERVING: *Choices/Exchanges 3 Lean Protein, ½ Fat; Calories 160 (from Fat 60); Fat 7g (Saturated 1.3g, Trans 0.0g); Cholesterol 50mg; Sodium 45mg; Potassium 180mg; Total Carbohydrate 2g (Dietary Fiber 0g, Sugars 0g); Protein 18g; Phosphorus 140mg.*

Grilled Lemon Mustard Chicken

PREP TIME: ABOUT 5 MIN PLUS MARINATING TIME	COOK TIME: 15 MIN	SERVINGS: 6	SERVING SIZE: 3 OUNCES

INGREDIENTS

Juice of 6 medium lemons

½ cup mustard seeds

1 tablespoon minced fresh tarragon

2 tablespoons freshly ground black pepper

4 garlic cloves, minced

2 tablespoons extra-virgin olive oil

Three 8-ounce boneless, skinless chicken breasts, halved

DIRECTIONS

1 In a small mixing bowl, combine the lemon juice, mustard seeds, tarragon, pepper, garlic, and oil; mix well.

2 Place the chicken in a baking dish, and pour the marinade on top. Cover, and refrigerate overnight.

3 Grill the chicken over medium heat for 10–15 minutes, basting with the marinade. Serve hot.

PER SERVING: *Choices/Exchanges ½ Carbohydrate, 4 Lean Protein, 1 Fat; Calories 260 (from Fat 120); Fat 13g (Saturated 1.7g, Trans 0.0g); Cholesterol 65mg; Sodium 70mg; Potassium 390mg; Total Carbohydrate 9g (Dietary Fiber 3g, Sugars 2g); Protein 28g; Phosphorus 310mg.*

Herbed Cornish Hens

PREP TIME: ABOUT 5 MIN PLUS MARINATING TIME	COOK TIME: 30 MIN	SERVINGS: 8	SERVING SIZE: ½ CORNISH HEN

INGREDIENTS

4 Cornish hens, giblets removed (about 1¼ pound each)

2 cups white wine, divided

2 garlic cloves, minced

1 small onion, minced

½ teaspoon celery seeds

½ teaspoon poultry seasoning

½ teaspoon paprika

½ teaspoon dried oregano

¼ teaspoon freshly ground black pepper

DIRECTIONS

1 Using a long, sharp knife, split each hen lengthwise. You may also buy precut hens.

2 Place the hens, cavity side up, on a rack in a shallow roasting pan. Pour 1½ cups of the wine over the hens; set aside.

3 In a shallow bowl, combine the garlic, onion, celery seeds, poultry seasoning, paprika, oregano, and pepper. Sprinkle half of the combined seasonings over the cavity of each split half. Cover, and refrigerate. Allow the hens to marinate for 2–3 hours.

4 Preheat the oven to 350 degrees. Bake the hens uncovered for 1 hour. Remove from the oven, turn breast side up, and remove the skin. Pour the remaining ½ cup of wine over the top, and sprinkle with the remaining seasonings.

5 Continue to bake for an additional 25–30 minutes, basting every 10 minutes until the hens are done. Transfer to a serving platter, and serve hot.

PER SERVING: *Choices/Exchanges 4 Lean Protein; Calories 190 (from Fat 45); Fat 5g (Saturated 1.2g, Trans 0.0g); Cholesterol 130mg; Sodium 80mg; Potassium 350mg; Total Carbohydrate 2g (Dietary Fiber 0g, Sugars 1g); Protein 29g; Phosphorus 195mg.*

Slow-Roasted Turkey Breast in Beer–Mustard Sauce

PREP TIME: ABOUT 5 MIN	COOK TIME: 2½ HR	SERVINGS: 10	SERVING SIZE: 3 OUNCES TURKEY

INGREDIENTS

5-pound, bone-in turkey breast, skin removed

1 tablespoon prepared mustard

½ cup light beer

¼ cup red wine vinegar

¾ cup ketchup

1 tablespoon no-added-salt tomato paste

½ cup spicy no-added-salt tomato juice (or spice up mild juice with several drops of hot pepper sauce)

¼ teaspoon freshly ground black pepper

DIRECTIONS

1 Preheat the oven to 350 degrees.

2 Spread the turkey breast with mustard.

3 In a small bowl, combine the beer, vinegar, ketchup, tomato paste, and tomato juice. Pour the mixture over the turkey, and then sprinkle with pepper.

4 Roast, covered, for 1½ hours at 350 degrees. Remove the cover, and roast an additional 1 hour, basting occasionally. Transfer to a serving platter, and serve.

PER SERVING: *Choices/Exchanges ½ Carbohydrate, 5 Lean Protein; Calories 220 (from Fat 25); Fat 3g (Saturated 0.8g, Trans 0.0g); Cholesterol 105mg; Sodium 350mg; Potassium 440mg; Total Carbohydrate 6g (Dietary Fiber 0g, Sugars 5g); Protein 39g; Phosphorus 310mg.*

Ginger Curry Chicken Kabobs

PREP TIME: ABOUT 5 MIN PLUS MARINATING TIME	COOK TIME: 5 MIN	SERVINGS: 4	SERVING SIZE: 3 OUNCES

INGREDIENTS

4 teaspoons fresh lemon juice

½ teaspoon cayenne pepper

¼ teaspoon freshly ground black pepper

1-inch piece of fresh ginger, peeled and minced

1 teaspoon curry powder

4 teaspoons extra-virgin olive oil

Two 8-ounce boneless, skinless chicken breasts, halved and cut into ¼-inch strips

DIRECTIONS

1 In a medium bowl, combine all ingredients except the chicken. Add the chicken, and let marinate overnight in the refrigerator.

2 Thread the chicken onto metal or wooden skewers (remember to soak the wooden skewers in water before using).

3 Grill over medium heat until the chicken is no longer pink, about 15 minutes. Transfer to a platter, and serve.

PER SERVING: *Choices/Exchanges 3 Lean Protein, ½ Fat; Calories 170 (from Fat 60); Fat 7g (Saturated 1.4g, Trans 0.0g); Cholesterol 65mg; Sodium 60mg; Potassium 220mg; Total Carbohydrate 1g (Dietary Fiber 0g, Sugars 0g); Protein 24g; Phosphorus 175mg.*

Oven-Baked Chicken Tenders

PREP TIME: ABOUT 5 MIN	COOK TIME: 12 MIN	SERVINGS: 4	SERVING SIZE: 3 OUNCES

INGREDIENTS

Two 8-ounce boneless, skinless chicken breasts, halved

2 egg whites, beaten

½ cup whole-wheat cracker crumbs

1 teaspoon paprika

2 teaspoons grated fresh Parmigiano-Reggiano cheese

DIRECTIONS

1 Preheat the oven to 350 degrees.

2 Cut each chicken breast into 2½-inch strips. Dip each strip into the egg whites.

3 On a flat plate or in a plastic bag, combine the cracker crumbs with paprika and cheese. Add the chicken strips, and coat with the crumb mixture.

4 On a nonstick cookie sheet, place the chicken strips side by side in one layer. Bake at 350 degrees for 10–12 minutes until golden and crunchy.

TIP: Kids will love these easy-to-eat strips of crunchy chicken that are baked, not fried. Serve with Marinara Sauce (see Chapter 6).

PER SERVING: *Choices/Exchanges ½ Starch, 4 Lean Protein; Calories 190 (from Fat 45); Fat 5g (Saturated 1.3g, Trans 0.0g); Cholesterol 65mg; Sodium 160mg; Potassium 280mg; Total Carbohydrate 9g (Dietary Fiber 1g, Sugars 1g); Protein 27g; Phosphorus 220mg.*

Wine-Poached Chicken with Herbs and Vegetables

PREP TIME: ABOUT 5 MIN	COOK TIME: 1 HR	SERVINGS: 8	SERVING SIZE: 3 OUNCES PLUS ½ CUP VEGETABLES

INGREDIENTS

4 quarts low-sodium chicken broth

2 cups dry white wine

4 large bay leaves

4 sprigs fresh thyme

¼ teaspoon freshly ground black pepper

4-pound chicken, giblets removed, washed and patted dry

½ pound carrots, peeled and julienned

½ pound turnips, peeled and julienned

½ pound parsnips, peeled and julienned

4 small leeks, washed and trimmed

DIRECTIONS

1 In a large stockpot, combine the broth, wine, bay leaves, thyme, dash salt (optional), and pepper. Let simmer over medium heat while you prepare the chicken.

2 Stuff the cavity with ⅓ each of the carrots, turnips, and parsnips; then truss. Add the stuffed chicken to the stockpot, and poach, covered, over low heat for 30 minutes.

3 Add the remaining vegetables with the leeks, and continue to simmer for 25–30 minutes, or until juices run clear when the chicken is pierced with a fork.

4 Remove the chicken and vegetables to a serving platter. Carve the chicken, remove the skin, and surround the sliced meat with poached vegetables to serve.

PER SERVING: *Choices/Exchanges 2 Nonstarchy Vegetable, 3 Lean Protein; Calories 190 (from Fat 45); Fat 5g (Saturated 1.5g, Trans 0.0g); Cholesterol 65mg; Sodium 105mg; Potassium 410mg; Total Carbohydrate 11g (Dietary Fiber 2g, Sugars 4g); Protein 23g; Phosphorus 160mg.*

Sautéed Chicken with Artichoke Hearts

PREP TIME: ABOUT 5 MIN	COOK TIME: 20 MIN	SERVINGS: 6	SERVING SIZE: 3–4 OUNCES WITH ½ CUP ARTICHOKES/SAUCE

INGREDIENTS

Nonstick cooking spray

Three 8-ounce boneless, skinless chicken breasts, halved

½ cup low-sodium chicken stock

¼ cup dry white wine

Two 8-ounce cans artichoke hearts, packed in water, drained and quartered

1 medium onion, diced

1 medium green bell pepper, chopped

2 tablespoons minced fresh tarragon or mint

¼ teaspoon white pepper

2 teaspoons cornstarch

1 tablespoon cold water

2 medium tomatoes, cut into wedges

DIRECTIONS

1 Coat a large skillet with nonstick cooking spray; place over medium heat until hot. Add the chicken, and sauté until lightly browned, about 3–4 minutes per side.

2 Add the chicken stock, wine, artichokes, onion, green pepper, tarragon or mint, and white pepper; stir well. Bring to a boil, cover, reduce heat, and let simmer for 10–15 minutes or until the chicken is no longer pink and the vegetables are just tender.

3 In a small bowl, combine the cornstarch and water; add to the chicken mixture along with the tomato wedges, stirring until the mixture has thickened. Remove from the heat, and serve.

VARY IT! Broccoli, asparagus, and bell peppers would also make great additions to this recipe.

PER SERVING: *Choices/Exchanges 2 Nonstarchy Vegetable, 3 Lean Protein; Calories 190 (from Fat 25); Fat 3g (Saturated 0.8g, Trans 0.0g); Cholesterol 65mg; Sodium 200mg; Potassium 540mg; Total Carbohydrate 12g (Dietary Fiber 4g, Sugars 3g); Protein 27g; Phosphorus 235mg.*

Spicy Chicken Drumsticks

PREP TIME: ABOUT 5 MIN PLUS MARINATING TIME	COOK TIME: 50 MIN	SERVINGS: 2	SERVING SIZE: 2 DRUMSTICKS

INGREDIENTS

¼ cup plain low-fat yogurt

2 tablespoons hot pepper sauce

Crushed red pepper flakes, to taste

4 chicken drumsticks, skinned (about 1 pound)

¼ cup dried bread crumbs

DIRECTIONS

1 In a shallow dish, combine the yogurt, hot pepper sauce, and crushed red pepper flakes, mixing well. Add the drumsticks, turning to coat. Cover, and marinate in the refrigerator for 2–4 hours.

2 Preheat the oven to 350 degrees.

3 Remove the drumsticks from the marinade, dredge in the bread crumbs, and place in a baking dish. Bake at 350 degrees for 40–50 minutes. Transfer to a serving platter, and serve.

PER SERVING: *Choices/Exchanges 1 Starch, 4 Lean Protein; Calories 250 (from Fat 60); Fat 7g (Saturated 1.9g, Trans 0.0g); Cholesterol 100mg; Sodium 290mg; Potassium 350mg; Total Carbohydrate 11g (Dietary Fiber 1g, Sugars 2g); Protein 33g; Phosphorus 250mg.*

Turkey Burgers

PREP TIME: ABOUT 5 MIN	COOK TIME: 15 MIN	SERVINGS: 6	SERVING SIZE: 3 OUNCES

INGREDIENTS

1¼ pounds ground turkey breast

1 egg white

1 tablespoon grated onion

¼ teaspoon dried thyme

½ teaspoon poultry seasoning

¼ teaspoon dried sage

Freshly ground black pepper

6 tablespoons Homemade Seasoned Bread Crumbs (see Chapter 14)

DIRECTIONS

1 In a medium bowl, combine all the ingredients except the bread crumbs. Form the meat into 6 patties, and press each one lightly into the bread crumbs.

2 Prepare an outside grill or oven broiler, and grill or broil 6 inches from the heat for 4–5 minutes per side until cooked through. Serve warm on split buns and with your favorite condiments.

PER SERVING: *Choices/Exchanges 3 Lean Protein; Calories 120 (from Fat 5); Fat 0.5g (Saturated 0.2g, Trans 0.0g); Cholesterol 60mg; Sodium 90mg; Potassium 240mg; Total Carbohydrate 3g (Dietary Fiber 0g, Sugars 0g); Protein 23g; Phosphorus 180mg.*

Turkey with Almond Duxelles

PREP TIME: ABOUT 5 MIN	COOK TIME: 30–40 MIN	SERVINGS: 8	SERVING SIZE: 1 TURKEY CUTLET PLUS SAUCE

INGREDIENTS

2 tablespoons extra-virgin olive oil

¼ cup dry sherry

¾ pound diced fresh mushrooms

4 medium shallots, finely minced

2 garlic cloves, minced

1 teaspoon minced fresh thyme

Dash cayenne pepper

½ cup ground almonds

¼ teaspoon freshly ground black pepper

2 pounds turkey breast cutlets, pounded to ¼-inch thickness and cut into 8 portions

Paprika, for garnish

½ cup low-fat plain Greek yogurt

DIRECTIONS

1 Preheat the oven to 350 degrees.

2 In a large skillet over medium heat, heat the olive oil and sherry. Add the mushrooms, shallots, garlic, thyme, and cayenne pepper. Cook, stirring often, until the mushrooms turn dark. Add the ground almonds, dash salt (optional), and pepper, and sauté for 2–3 minutes.

3 Divide the mixture into 8 portions, and place each portion in the center of each turkey portion. Fold the edges over, roll up, and place in a baking dish, seam side down, 1 inch apart.

4 Place about 1 tablespoon Greek yogurt over each turkey roll, and sprinkle with paprika. Bake at 350 degrees for 25–30 minutes or until the turkey is tender. Transfer to a serving platter, and serve.

PER SERVING: *CHOICES/EXCHANGES ½ Carbohydrate, 4 Lean Protein, ½ Fat; Calories 240 (from Fat 90); Fat 10g (Saturated 1.5g, Trans 0.0g); Cholesterol 70mg; Sodium 100mg; Potassium 480mg; Total Carbohydrate 6g (Dietary Fiber 2g, Sugars 2g); Protein 32g; Phosphorus 310mg.*

Chapter 8

Beef, Pork, Lamb, and Veal

RECIPES IN THIS CHAPTER

Apple Cinnamon Pork Chops

Creole Steak

Beef and Vegetable Shish Kabobs

Butterflied Beef Eye Roast

Herbed Chipotle Pot Roast

Lamb Chops with Orange Sauce

Marinated Leg of Lamb

Marvelous Meat Loaf

Pork Chops Milanese

Spice-Infused Roast Beef

Pork Tenderloin Stir-Fry

Quinoa-Stuffed Peppers

Veal Romano

Veal Scaloppine

Beef, pork, lamb, and veal are hearty and delicious protein options, but they're generally higher in saturated fat than other types of protein such as poultry and fish. People with diabetes can enjoy red meats and pork, but they should eat these proteins in moderation and try to choose the leanest, highest-quality cuts available.

The recipes in this chapter will demonstrate a variety of ways to prepare lean cuts of red meat and pork so you can enjoy savory, meat-based entrées without jeopardizing your healthy eating goals.

TIP

Trimming excess fat from meat before cooking is a great way to reduce the fat content of your meal; many of the recipes in this chapter employ this technique.

These diabetes-friendly dishes are full of rich flavors. All the recipes in this chapter are easy enough to prepare on a busy weeknight, but special enough for entertaining. Even if you're already an expert at preparing healthy beef and pork at home, you'll be pleased to find a few simple, elegant lamb and veal recipes in the pages ahead that are sure to impress your friends and family! These healthy, delicious recipes will turn any night into a special occasion.

Apple Cinnamon Pork Chops

PREP TIME: ABOUT 5 MIN	COOK TIME: 20 MIN	SERVINGS: 2	SERVING SIZE: 1 PORK CHOP WITH APPLES

INGREDIENTS

2 teaspoons extra-virgin olive oil

1 large apple, sliced

½ teaspoon organic cinnamon

⅛ teaspoon freshly grated nutmeg

Two 3-ounce lean boneless pork chops, trimmed of fat

DIRECTIONS

1 In a medium nonstick skillet, heat the olive oil. Add the apple slices, and sauté until just tender. Sprinkle with cinnamon and nutmeg, remove from heat, and keep warm.

2 Place the pork chops in the skillet, and cook thoroughly; a meat thermometer inserted into the thickest part of the meat should reach 145 degrees. Remove the pork chops from the skillet, arrange on a serving platter, spoon the apple slices on top, and serve.

TIP: Cinnamon is beneficial in regulating blood sugar levels. Consider serving this dish with baked sweet potatoes or quinoa, also sprinkled with cinnamon.

VARY IT! Chicken and turkey also work well in this recipe.

PER SERVING: *Choices/Exchanges 1 Fruit, 2 Lean Protein, 1 Fat; Calories 210 (from Fat 90); Fat 10g (Saturated 2.6g, Trans 0.0g); Cholesterol 45mg; Sodium 35mg; Potassium 340mg; Total Carbohydrate 15g (Dietary Fiber 3g, Sugars 11g); Protein 16g; Phosphorus 145mg.*

Creole Steak

PREP TIME: ABOUT 5 MIN | COOK TIME: 1 HR 40 MIN | SERVINGS: 4 | SERVING SIZE: 3 OUNCES

INGREDIENTS

2 teaspoons extra-virgin olive oil

¼ cup chopped onion

¼ cup chopped green bell pepper

1 cup canned crushed tomatoes

½ teaspoon chili powder

¼ teaspoon celery seed

4 cloves garlic, finely chopped

¼ teaspoon salt

1 teaspoon cumin

1 pound lean boneless round steak

DIRECTIONS

1 In a large skillet over medium heat, heat the oil. Add the onions and green pepper, and sauté until the onions are translucent (about 5 minutes).

2 Add the tomatoes, chili powder, celery seed, garlic, salt, and cumin; cover and let simmer over low heat for 20–25 minutes. This allows the flavors to blend.

3 Preheat the oven to 350 degrees. Trim all visible fat off the steak.

4 In a nonstick pan or a pan that has been sprayed with nonstick cooking spray, lightly brown the steak on each side. Transfer the steak to a 13-x-9-x-2-inch baking dish; pour the sauce over the steak, and cover.

5 Bake for 1¼ hours or until the steak is tender. Remove from the oven; slice the steak, and arrange on a serving platter. Spoon the sauce over the steak, and serve.

VARY IT! Lamb would also work well in this recipe. Serve with brown rice or mashed cauliflower.

TIP: In addition to its great flavor, cumin is also known for its anti-inflammatory properties. Because inflammation plays a role in illness, reducing it can lead to better overall health.

PER SERVING: *Choices/Exchanges 1 Nonstarchy Vegetable, 4 Lean Protein; Calories 200 (from Fat 50); Fat 6g (Saturated 1.6g, Trans 0.0g); Cholesterol 50mg; Sodium 270mg; Potassium 450mg; Total Carbohydrate 7g (Dietary Fiber 2g, Sugars 3g); Protein 28g; Phosphorus 195mg.*

Beef and Vegetable Shish Kabobs

PREP TIME: ABOUT 15 MIN PLUS MARINATING TIME	COOK TIME: 20 MIN	SERVINGS: 8	SERVING SIZE: 1 KABOB (2 OUNCES BEEF) PLUS VEGETABLES

INGREDIENTS

2 teaspoons canola oil

¼ cup red wine vinegar

1 tablespoon light soy sauce

4 garlic cloves, minced

2 tablespoons freshly squeezed lemon juice

⅛ teaspoon freshly ground black pepper

1½ pounds boneless beef top sirloin steak, cut into 24 cubes

2 large bell peppers, red and green, cut into 1-inch pieces

1 pound mushrooms, stemmed

1 large tomato, cut into wedges

1 medium onion, quartered

DIRECTIONS

1 In a small bowl, combine the oil, vinegar, soy sauce, garlic, lemon juice, and pepper. Pour over the beef cubes, and let marinate in the refrigerator 3–4 hours or overnight.

2 Place 3 beef cubes on 8 metal or wooden skewers (remember to soak the wooden skewers in water before using), alternating with peppers, mushroom caps, tomato wedges, and onions.

3 Grill over medium heat, turning often and basting with marinade until the meat is cooked through. Arrange the skewers on a platter to serve.

TIP: While the kabobs are cooking, simmer some rice, and add a salad for a complete meal.

VARY IT! You could use chicken and/or lamb in this recipe.

PER SERVING: Choices/Exchanges 2 Nonstarchy Vegetable, 2 Lean Protein; Calories 150 (from Fat 40); Fat 4.5g (Saturated 1.4g, Trans 0.1g); Cholesterol 30mg; Sodium 110mg; Potassium 550mg; Total Carbohydrate 8g (Dietary Fiber 2g, Sugars 4g); Protein 19g; Phosphorus 200mg.

Butterflied Beef Eye Roast

PREP TIME: ABOUT 10 MIN PLUS MARINATING TIME	COOK TIME: 40 MIN	SERVINGS: 12	SERVING SIZE: 3–4 OUNCES

INGREDIENTS

3-pound lean beef eye roast

3 tablespoons extra-virgin olive oil

¼ cup water

½ cup red wine vinegar

3 garlic cloves, minced

½ teaspoon crushed red pepper

1 tablespoon chopped fresh thyme

DIRECTIONS

1 Slice the roast down the middle, open it, and lay it flat in a shallow baking dish.

2 In a small bowl, combine the remaining ingredients, and pour the mixture over the roast. Cover, and let the meat marinate in the refrigerator for at least 12 hours, or up to 24 hours. Turn the roast occasionaly.

3 Set the oven to broil. Remove the roast from the marinade, discard the marinade, and place the roast on a rack in the broiler pan. Broil the roast 5–7 inches from the heat, turning occasionally, for 20–25 minutes or until desired degree of doneness.

4 Remove from the oven, cover with foil, and let stand for 15–20 minutes before carving. Transfer to a serving platter, spoon any juices over the top, and serve.

VARY IT! Veal shoulder and leg of lamb can also be prepared this way.

TIP: Pureed squash and broccoli would make great accompaniments to this dish.

PER SERVING: *Choices/Exchanges 4 Lean Protein; Calories 160 (from Fat 45); Fat 5g (Saturated 1.5g, Trans 0.0g); Cholesterol 50mg; Sodium 35mg; Potassium 220mg; Total Carbohydrate 0g (Dietary Fiber 0g, Sugars 0g); Protein 26g; Phosphorus 165mg.*

Herbed Chipotle Pot Roast

PREP TIME: ABOUT 5 MIN	COOK TIME: 3 HR	SERVINGS: 8	SERVING SIZE: 3 OUNCES

INGREDIENTS

1 tablespoon extra-virgin olive oil

One 2-pound lean boneless beef roast

⅛ teaspoon freshly ground black pepper

½ cup water

⅓ cup dry sherry

¼ cup chipotle sauce

1 garlic clove, minced

¼ teaspoon dried rosemary

¼ teaspoon dried thyme

2 medium onions, sliced

1 bay leaf

1 cup sliced mushrooms

DIRECTIONS

1 Add the olive oil to a large Dutch oven over medium heat. Sprinkle the roast with the pepper; brown the roast on all sides.

2 Combine the water, sherry, chipotle, garlic, rosemary, and thyme in a small bowl, and pour over the roast. Add the onions and bay leaf, cover, and simmer for 2–3 hours, until the roast is tender.

3 During the last 15 minutes, add the mushrooms, and continue simmering until heated. Remove the bay leaf. Transfer the roast to a platter, slice, and serve.

TIP: Serve this mouthwatering roast with Colorful Rice Casserole or Asian Fried Rice (see Chapter 13).

PER SERVING: *Choices/Exchanges 1 Nonstarchy Vegetable, 3 Lean Protein, ½ Fat; Calories 180 (from Fat 70); Fat 8g (Saturated 2.1g, Trans 0.2g); Cholesterol 70mg; Sodium 95mg; Potassium 360mg; Total Carbohydrate 5g (Dietary Fiber 1g, Sugars 2g); Protein 23g; Phosphorus 190mg.*

Lamb Chops with Orange Sauce

PREP TIME: ABOUT 5 MIN PLUS MARINATING TIME	COOK TIME: 20 MIN	SERVINGS: 4	SERVING SIZE: 2 LAMB CHOPS WITH SAUCE

INGREDIENTS

½ cup freshly squeezed orange juice

2 tablespoons orange zest

1 teaspoon fresh or ½ teaspoon dried thyme

⅛ teaspoon freshly ground black pepper

Nonstick cooking spray

8 small lean lamb chops, about ½ inch thick (about 4 ounces each)

1 cup sliced fresh mushrooms

½ cup dry white wine

DIRECTIONS

1 In a shallow baking dish, combine the orange juice, orange zest, thyme, and pepper; mix well.

2 Trim all excess fat from the lamb chops and place in a baking dish. Spoon the orange juice mixture over the chops; cover, and refrigerate for 3–4 hours, occasionally turning chops.

3 Coat a large skillet with nonstick cooking spray; place over medium-high heat until hot. Remove the chops from the marinade, reserving the marinade; arrange in the skillet. Brown the chops on both sides, remove from the skillet, and set on a plate lined with paper towels.

4 Reduce the heat to medium, add the mushrooms, and sauté until just tender. Stir in the reserved marinade and wine, and bring to a boil.

5 Return the lamb chops to the skillet; cover, reduce heat, and simmer for 10–12 minutes or until the sauce is reduced to about ½ cup. Transfer the lamb chops to a platter, spoon the orange sauce on top, and serve.

TIP: Try serving these delicious orange lamb chops with baby peas or French green beans.

PER SERVING: *Choices/Exchanges ½ Carbohydrate, 4 Lean Protein, ½ Fat; Calories 250 (from Fat 90); Fat 10g (Saturated 3.5g, Trans 0.0g); Cholesterol 95mg; Sodium 85mg; Potassium 510mg; Total Carbohydrate 5g (Dietary Fiber 1g, Sugars 3g); Protein 31g; Phosphorus 250mg.*

Marinated Leg of Lamb

PREP TIME: ABOUT 5 MIN PLUS MARINATING TIME	COOK TIME: 40 MIN	SERVINGS: 16	SERVING SIZE: 3½–4 OUNCES

INGREDIENTS

1 leg of lamb (7 pounds including bone), boned, butterflied, and visible fat removed

3 cups dry red wine

¼ cup extra-virgin olive oil

2 medium onions, sliced

1 large carrot, thinly sliced

6 parsley sprigs

2 bay leaves, crumbled

4 cloves garlic, minced

⅛ teaspoon freshly ground black pepper

Fresh parsley sprigs

DIRECTIONS

1 In a large ceramic, glass, or stainless steel dish (anything but plastic), combine all the ingredients except the parsley sprigs; cover, refrigerate, and let marinate for 1–2 days, turning occasionally.

2 After marinating, drain the lamb, discard the marinade, and pat dry. Season with salt, if desired. Place the lamb into a grill basket. Broil the lamb 3–4 inches from the heat for 15–20 minutes per side.

3 Transfer the lamb to a cutting board and let cool slightly. Carve the lamb diagonally; transfer to a serving platter, garnish with parsley sprigs, and serve.

TIP: Marinating 1–2 days is the secret to a great leg of lamb. Serve with sautéed carrots and oven-roasted potatoes.

PER SERVING: *Choices/Exchanges 4 Lean Protein; Calories 200 (from Fat 70); Fat 8g (Saturated 3.2g, Trans 0.0g); Cholesterol 90mg; Sodium 75mg; Potassium 350mg; Total Carbohydrate 0g (Dietary Fiber 0g, Sugars 0g); Protein 29g; Phosphorus 230mg.*

Marvelous Meat Loaf

PREP TIME: ABOUT 15 MIN | COOK TIME: 2 HR | SERVINGS: 10 | SERVING SIZE: 3 OUNCES

INGREDIENTS

1 pound 95 percent lean ground beef

1 pound ground turkey breast

¾ cup Homemade Seasoned Bread Crumbs (see Chapter 14)

½ cup fat-free milk

2 egg whites

1 medium onion, finely chopped

1 bunch fresh cilantro or parsley, or a combination of both, finely chopped

⅛ teaspoon freshly ground black pepper

One 14.5-ounce can fire-roasted tomatoes

DIRECTIONS

1 Preheat the oven to 350 degrees.

2 In a large bowl, combine all ingredients except the tomatoes, and form into a loaf.

3 Place into a loaf pan and bake at 350 degrees for 1¼–1½ hours, until internal temperature registers 165 degrees.

4 Pour the tomatoes over the top during the last 20 minutes of baking.

5 Remove from the oven, cover with foil, and let stand for 10 minutes before serving.

VARY IT! For variety, you can add ¼ cup shredded carrot, 2 tablespoons chopped green pepper, and/or ¼ cup sliced celery in Step 2.

PER SERVING: *Exchanges ½ Carbohydrate; 3 Lean Protein; Calories 160 (from Fat 30); Fat 3.5g (Saturated 1.3g, Trans 0.1g); Cholesterol 55mg; Sodium 220mg; Potassium 480mg; Total Carbohydrate 7g (Dietary Fiber 1g; Sugars 3g); Protein 23g; Phosphorus 235mg.*

Pork Chops Milanese

PREP TIME: ABOUT 5 MIN	COOK TIME: 20 MIN	SERVINGS: 4	SERVING SIZE: 1 PORK CHOP

INGREDIENTS

¾ cup Homemade Seasoned Bread Crumbs (see Chapter 14)

1 tablespoon Parmigiano-Reggiano cheese

Four 3-ounce lean boneless pork chops, trimmed of fat

1 egg and ¼ cup water, slightly beaten

1 tablespoon extra-virgin olive oil

2 large lemons, cut into wedges

DIRECTIONS

1 In a shallow bowl, combine the bread crumbs and Parmigiano-Reggiano cheese.

2 Dip the pork chops in the egg mixture, and dredge in the bread crumb mixture.

3 In a large nonstick skillet, heat the olive oil. Add the pork chops and brown on both sides. Reduce the heat, cover, and sauté for 3–5 minutes. Remove cover, and cook 5–10 minutes more until the pork is no longer pink, and a meat thermometer inserted in the thickest part of the meat reads 145 degrees.

4 Squeeze 2 or 3 lemon wedges over the chops. Transfer to a serving platter, garnish with the remaining lemon wedges, and serve.

VARY IT! Chicken, turkey, veal, beef, and fish fillets can also be prepared this way.

PER SERVING: *Choices/Exchanges ½ Starch, 3 Lean Protein, ½ Fat; Calories 200 (from Fat 100); Fat 11g (Saturated 3.0g, Trans 0.0g); Cholesterol 90mg; Sodium 170mg; Potassium 280mg; Total Carbohydrate 8g (Dietary Fiber 1g, Sugars 1g); Protein 19g; Phosphorus 190mg.*

Spice-Infused Roast Beef

PREP TIME: ABOUT 5 MIN	COOK TIME: 1½ HR	SERVINGS: 8	SERVING SIZE: 3 OUNCES

INGREDIENTS

¾ cup grated onion, divided

1 tablespoon caraway seeds

1 teaspoon ground coriander

1 teaspoon ground ginger

2-pound lean boneless chuck roast

1 tablespoon extra-virgin olive oil

⅓ cup red wine vinegar

1 cup unsweetened apple juice

1 bunch fresh parsley, minced

DIRECTIONS

1 Preheat the oven to 325 degrees.

2 In a small bowl, combine ¼ cup of the onion, caraway seeds, coriander, and ginger, and rub into the roast.

3 In a medium saucepan over medium heat, sauté the remaining ½ cup of onion in olive oil. Place the roast in a roasting pan, and add the sautéed onion.

4 Add the vinegar, apple juice, parsley, and ½ cup water to the roasting pan. Bake the roast uncovered at 325 degrees for 1–1½ hours, basting frequently. Transfer the roast to a platter, and slice.

TIP: Serve this hearty dish with cabbage and noodles.

PER SERVING: *Choices/Exchanges ½ Carbohydrate, 3 Lean Protein; Calories 190 (from Fat 70); Fat 8g (Saturated 2.1g, Trans 0.2g); Cholesterol 70mg; Sodium 50mg; Potassium 380mg; Total Carbohydrate 6g (Dietary Fiber 1g, Sugars 4g); Protein 23g; Phosphorus 185mg.*

Pork Tenderloin Stir-Fry

PREP TIME: ABOUT 5 MIN	COOK TIME: 20 MIN	SERVINGS: 6	SERVING SIZE: 3.5 OUNCES

INGREDIENTS

1 tablespoon sesame oil

1-pound pork tenderloin, cut into thin strips

1 tablespoon oyster sauce (found in the Asian food section of the grocery store)

1 tablespoon cornstarch

½ cup low-sodium chicken broth

1 tablespoon light soy sauce

1 cup fresh snow peas, trimmed

1 cup broccoli florets

½ cup sliced water chestnuts, drained

1 cup diced red pepper

¼ cup sliced scallions

DIRECTIONS

1 In a large skillet or wok, heat the oil. Stir-fry the pork until the strips are no longer pink.

2 In a measuring cup, combine the oyster sauce, cornstarch, chicken broth, and soy sauce. Add the sauce to the pork, and cook until the sauce thickens.

3 Add the vegetables, cover, and steam for 5 minutes. Serve.

PER SERVING: *Choices/Exchanges 1 Nonstarchy Vegetable, 2 Lean Protein, ½ Fat; Calories 130 (from Fat 40); Fat 4.5g (Saturated 1.0g, Trans 0.0g); Cholesterol 40mg; Sodium 210mg; Potassium 400mg; Total Carbohydrate 7g (Dietary Fiber 2g, Sugars 2g); Protein 16g; Phosphorus 165mg.*

Quinoa-Stuffed Peppers

PREP TIME: ABOUT 15 MIN	COOK TIME: 45 MIN	SERVINGS: 4	SERVING SIZE: 1 PEPPER

INGREDIENTS

4 medium bell peppers, red or green (or both)

1 pound lean ground sirloin

1 small onion, minced

⅔ cup cooked quinoa

1 cup sautéed spinach

¼ cup chopped fresh oregano or cilantro

⅛ teaspoon salt

⅛ teaspoon freshly ground black pepper

One 8-ounce can tomato sauce, divided

¼ cup pinot noir or chianti

DIRECTIONS

1 Slice off the stem end of each pepper, and remove the seeds.

2 In a medium bowl, combine the beef, onion, quinoa, spinach, oregano, salt, pepper, and ⅓ cup tomato sauce; mix well. Stuff the mixture into the peppers, and place them in a medium saucepan. Pour the wine and remaining tomato sauce over the peppers.

3 Bring the peppers to a boil; cover, and let simmer until tender, about 45 minutes. Add a few tablespoons of water if the sauce begins to cook away. Transfer to a serving platter, drizzle the remaining sauce over the top, and serve.

VARY IT! You can use this basic filling to stuff zucchini or yellow squash, too.

PER SERVING: *Choices/Exchanges ½ Starch, 3 Nonstarchy Vegetable, 4 Lean Protein; Calories 280 (from Fat 50); Fat 6g (Saturated 1.7g, Trans 0.2g); Cholesterol 80mg; Sodium 460mg; Potassium 1260mg; Total Carbohydrate 23g (Dietary Fiber 6g, Sugars 9g); Protein 31g; Phosphorus 385mg.*

Veal Romano

PREP TIME: ABOUT 10 MIN | COOK TIME: 20 MIN | SERVINGS: 6 | SERVING SIZE: 3–4 OUNCES

INGREDIENTS

1½ pounds lean veal cutlets

¼ cup flour

2 tablespoons extra-virgin olive oil, divided

⅛ teaspoon freshly ground black pepper

½ cup dry white wine

½ cup roasted red peppers, drained and julienned

8 large black olives, thinly sliced

2 tablespoons capers, rinsed and drained

DIRECTIONS

1 Place the cutlets between two pieces of wax paper or on a cutting board, and pound with a meat hammer until they're about ¼ inch thick.

2 Lightly flour the veal, shaking off the excess. In a large, wide, nonstick skillet, heat 1 tablespoon of the olive oil over high heat.

3 Sauté the veal for 2–3 minutes on each side, transfer to a platter, and sprinkle with pepper. Continue until all veal is cooked. Set aside.

4 Add the remaining 1 tablespoon of olive oil to the skillet. Add the wine, and scrape the brown bits from the skillet. Reduce the heat to medium, and add the red peppers, olives, and capers, stirring occasionally.

5 Add the veal back to the pan. Continue cooking until heated through. Spoon the sauce over the veal and serve.

VARY IT! Chicken and cod filets taste great when prepared this way as well.

PER SERVING: *Choices/Exchanges ½ Carbohydrate, 4 Lean Protein; Calories 210 (from Fat 80); Fat 9g (Saturated 1.7g, Trans 0.0g); Cholesterol 80mg; Sodium 220mg; Potassium 380mg; Total Carbohydrate 6g (Dietary Fiber 1g, Sugars 1g); Protein 26g; Phosphorus 230mg.*

Veal Scaloppine

PREP TIME: ABOUT 10 MIN	COOK TIME: 20 MIN	SERVINGS: 4	SERVING SIZE: 3-4 OUNCES

INGREDIENTS

Four 4-ounce lean veal cutlets

⅛ teaspoon freshly ground black pepper

1 tablespoon extra-virgin olive oil

½ pound fresh mushrooms, sliced

1 large green bell pepper, cut into ½-inch strips

½ cup dry white wine

⅓ cup low-sodium chicken stock

1 tablespoon lemon juice

1 tablespoon cornstarch, combined with 2 tablespoons water, and stirred well to combine

2 tablespoons minced fresh parsley

DIRECTIONS

1 Place the veal cutlets between two pieces of wax paper, and pound until the cutlets are ⅛ inch thick. Sprinkle the veal with pepper, and set aside.

2 Heat the oil in a large skillet over medium heat. Add the veal, a few pieces at a time, cooking 2–3 minutes per side or until lightly browned. Remove from the skillet, place on a platter, and keep the veal warm while you prepare the sauce.

3 Sauté the mushrooms and green pepper in the skillet for 5 minutes or until tender. Add the wine, stock, and lemon juice and bring to a boil. Add the cornstarch mixture to the skillet, stirring constantly until the mixture has thickened.

4 Remove from the heat and stir in the parsley. Arrange the veal on a serving platter, and pour the sauce over the top.

TIP: Serve this classic dish with vermicelli and steamed broccoli or green beans.

VARY IT! You can substitute veal for chicken or beef in this recipe.

PER SERVING: *Choices/Exchanges 1 Nonstarchy Vegetable, 4 Lean Protein; Calories 200 (from Fat 50); Fat 6g (Saturated 1.3g, Trans 0.0g); Cholesterol 80mg; Sodium 85mg; Potassium 630mg; Total Carbohydrate 6g (Dietary Fiber 1g, Sugars 2g); Protein 28g; Phosphorus 285mg.*

Chapter 9

Seafood

RECIPES IN THIS CHAPTER

You don't have to visit the coast to enjoy delicious seafood dishes! The recipes in this chapter will help you fit rich, tasty seafood into your everyday diabetes meal plan. Fish and other kinds of seafood are a relatively lean type of protein, which makes them a good choice for people with diabetes; fish that contain omega-3 fatty acids (a "healthy" fat) are especially good options. However, when most people think of eating seafood, they probably picture battered, fried fish and shrimp or lobster soaked in melted butter. These kinds of seafood dishes are luxurious, but they can add a lot of unhealthy saturated fat to your diet. Try to avoid breaded and fried seafood and heavy sauces when choosing seafood options.

Luckily, there are healthier ways to prepare seafood that provide tons of flavor without adding to your waistline! Steamed, baked, grilled, and roasted seafood are great alternatives to traditional, fat-laden seafood dishes. Whether you're looking for a quick and easy dinner like Savory Boiled Shrimp (see the recipe later in this chapter), a grilled fish dish for your summer barbecue, or an elegant seafood entrée for a special occasion, this chapter has a healthy recipe for you!

WARNING

Fish are generally a good lean protein choice, but some types of fish have a high mercury content and should be enjoyed in moderation or, in some cases, avoided all together (especially by pregnant and breastfeeding women and small children). Fish choices with the highest mercury content include bigeye tuna, king mackerel, marlin, orange roughy, shark, swordfish, and tilefish. For more information, check out the Food and Drug Administration and Environmental Protection Agency's consumer advisories about fish available at www.fda.gov/downloads/Food/FoodborneIllnessContaminants/Metals/UCM537120.pdf.

Roasted Red Snapper and Shrimp in Parchment

PREP TIME: ABOUT 10 MIN	COOK TIME: 45 MIN	SERVINGS: 8	SERVING SIZE: 3 OUNCES

INGREDIENTS

One 3-pound whole red snapper or bass, cleaned

1 medium garlic clove, minced

¼ cup extra-virgin olive oil

⅛ teaspoon freshly ground black pepper

½ teaspoon finely chopped fresh thyme

1 teaspoon flour

½ pound large shrimp, shelled and deveined

½ pound sliced mushrooms

3 tablespoons lemon juice, divided

½ cup dry white wine, divided

¼ cup minced fresh parsley

Zest of 1 lemon

DIRECTIONS

1 Preheat oven to 375 degrees. Wash the fish, inside and out, under cold running water, and pat dry with paper towels.

2 In a small bowl, combine the garlic, olive oil, pepper, thyme, and flour. Mix well.

3 Place the fish on a double thickness of parchment paper. In the cavity of the fish, place 1 tablespoon of the garlic mixture, 4 shrimp, and ½ cup sliced mushrooms. Sprinkle with 1 tablespoon of the lemon juice and 2 tablespoons of the wine.

4 Dot the top of the fish with the remaining garlic mixture, and arrange the remaining shrimp and mushrooms on top. Sprinkle with the remaining lemon juice and wine, and the parsley.

5 Bring the long sides of the parchment together over the fish, and secure with a double fold. Fold both ends of the parchment upward several times.

6 Place the fish on a baking sheet; bake for 30–35 minutes at 375 degrees. Transfer to a serving platter, garnish with lemon zest, and serve.

VARY IT! Salmon and tuna filets also work well in this recipe.

TIP: If possible, use fresh (never frozen) shrimp or shrimp that are free of preservatives — for example, shrimp that haven't been treated with salt or sodium tripolyphosphate (STPP).

PER SERVING: *Choices/Exchanges 3 Lean Protein, ½ Fat; Calories 160 (from Fat 70); Fat 8g (Saturated 1.0g, Trans 0.0g); Cholesterol 55mg; Sodium 65mg; Potassium 440mg; Total Carbohydrate 2g (Dietary Fiber 0g, Sugars 1g); Protein 19g; Phosphorus 200mg.*

Baked Garlic Scampi

PREP TIME: ABOUT 5 MIN	COOK TIME: 10 MIN	SERVINGS: 4	SERVING SIZE: 3 OUNCES AND ½ CUP ARUGULA

INGREDIENTS

1 tablespoon extra-virgin olive oil

¼ teaspoon salt

7 garlic cloves, crushed

2 tablespoons chopped fresh parsley, divided

1 pound large shrimp, shelled (with tails left on) and deveined

Juice and zest of 1 lemon

2 cups baby arugula

DIRECTIONS

1 Preheat the oven to 350 degrees. Grease a 13-x-9-x-2-inch baking pan with the olive oil. Add the salt, garlic, and 1 table-spoon of the parsley in a medium bowl; mix well, and set aside.

2 Arrange the shrimp in a single layer in the baking pan, and bake for 3 minutes, uncovered. Turn the shrimp, and sprinkle with the lemon peel, lemon juice, and the remaining 1 table-spoon of parsley. Continue to bake 1–2 minutes more until the shrimp are bright pink and tender.

3 Remove the shrimp from the oven. Place the arugula on a serving platter, and top with the shrimp. Spoon the garlic mixture over the shrimp and arugula, and serve.

TIP: If possible, use fresh (never frozen) shrimp or shrimp that are free of preservatives — for example, shrimp that have not been treated with salt or sodium tripolyphosphate (STPP).

PER SERVING: *Choices/Exchanges 2 Lean Protein; Calories 110 (from Fat 30); Fat 3.5g (Saturated 0.5g, Trans 0.0g); Cholesterol 120mg; Sodium 220mg; Potassium 250mg; Total Carbohydrate 3g (Dietary Fiber 0g, Sugars 1g); Protein 16g; Phosphorus 165mg.*

Shrimp and Mushroom Casserole with Sherry Cream Sauce

PREP TIME: ABOUT 5 MIN	COOK TIME: 25–30 MIN	SERVINGS: 8	SERVING SIZE: 2½–3 OUNCES

INGREDIENTS

3 tablespoons extra-virgin olive oil, divided

1 pound mushrooms, sliced

2 tablespoons flour

½ teaspoon salt

⅛ teaspoon freshly ground black pepper

⅛ teaspoon nutmeg

1 cup plain fat-free yogurt

2 pounds shrimp (fresh, never frozen, preservative-free), shelled, deveined, and boiled for 2 minutes

½ cup dry sherry

½ cup Homemade Seasoned Bread Crumbs (see Chapter 14)

2 tablespoons chopped almonds

2 tablespoons chopped fresh parsley

DIRECTIONS

1 Preheat the oven to 350 degrees.

2 In a large nonstick skillet over medium heat, heat 1 tablespoon of olive oil. Add the mushrooms, and sauté for 3–5 minutes. With a slotted spoon, remove the mushrooms, and arrange on the bottom of a 1½-quart baking dish.

3 Add the remaining 2 tablespoons of olive oil to the skillet. Whisk in the flour, salt, pepper, and nutmeg until smooth. Gradually add the yogurt, stirring constantly. Reduce heat, and simmer until thickened.

4 Add the shrimp and sherry, mixing well. Spoon the shrimp mixture over the mushrooms in the baking dish. Mix the bread crumbs and almonds; sprinkle over the shrimp, and top with parsley.

5 Bake uncovered for 20 minutes at 350 degrees or until the casserole is heated through and bubbly. Remove from the oven, and serve hot.

TIP: If possible, use fresh (never frozen) shrimp or shrimp that are free of preservatives — for example, shrimp that have not been treated with salt or sodium tripolyphosphate (STPP).

PER SERVING: *Choices/Exchanges ½ Carbohydrate, 3 Lean Protein; Calories 170 (from Fat 50); Fat 6g (Saturated 0.9g, Trans 0.0g); Cholesterol 120mg; Sodium 280mg; Potassium 440mg; Total Carbohydrate 8g (Dietary Fiber 1g, Sugars 3g); Protein 19g; Phosphorus 265mg.*

Savory Boiled Shrimp

PREP TIME: ABOUT 5 MIN PLUS CHILLING TIME	COOK TIME: 10 MIN	SERVINGS: 6	SERVING SIZE: 4 OUNCES

INGREDIENTS

4 bay leaves

2 teaspoons Herbes de Provence or seafood seasoning

8 cups water

1 large lemon, quartered

1 garlic clove, minced

2 pounds large shrimp, shelled and deveined

DIRECTIONS

1 In a double or triple thickness of cheesecloth, combine the spices. Secure the packet with a piece of string.

2 Combine the water, lemon, garlic, and spice bag together in a Dutch oven. Bring the water to a boil, reduce the heat, and simmer for 3 minutes.

3 Add the shrimp, and return to a boil. Boil the shrimp for 3–5 minutes. Drain thoroughly, bring to room temperature, and then chill in the refrigerator. Serve with cocktail sauce, if desired.

VARY IT! These shrimp taste great tossed with pasta or vegetable noodles as well.

TIP: If possible use fresh (never frozen) shrimp or shrimp that are free of preservatives — for example, shrimp that have not been treated with salt or sodium tripolyphosphate (STPP).

PER SERVING: *Choices/Exchanges 2 Lean Protein; Calories 80 (from Fat 0); Fat 0g (Saturated 0.0g, Trans 0.0g); Cholesterol 160mg; Sodium 95mg; Potassium 220mg; Total Carbohydrate 0g (Dietary Fiber 0g, Sugars 0g); Protein 20g; Phosphorus 205mg.*

Broiled Sole with Mustard Sauce

PREP TIME: ABOUT 5 MIN	COOK TIME: 20 MIN	SERVINGS: 6	SERVING SIZE: 3 OUNCES WITH SAUCE

INGREDIENTS

Nonstick cooking spray

1½ pound fresh sole filets

3 tablespoons low-fat mayonnaise

2 tablespoons Dijon mustard

2 tablespoons chopped parsley

⅛ teaspoon freshly ground black pepper

1 large lemon, cut into wedges

DIRECTIONS

1 Preheat broiler. Coat a baking sheet with nonstick cooking spray. Arrange the filets so they don't overlap.

2 In a small bowl, combine the mayonnaise, mustard, parsley, and pepper, and mix thoroughly. Spread the mixture evenly over the filets. Broil 3–4 inches from the heat for 4 minutes until the fish flakes easily with a fork.

3 Arrange the filets on a serving platter, garnish with lemon wedges, and serve.

TIP: Try this recipe over blanched broccoli or string beans.

VARY IT! Chicken and salmon fillets work well with this recipe, too.

PER SERVING: *Exchanges 3 Lean Protein; Calories 120 (from Fat 20); Fat 2g (Saturated 0.4g, Trans 0.0g); Cholesterol 60 mg; Sodium 280mg; Potassium 330mg; Total Carbohydrate 2g (Dietary Fiber 0g, Sugars 1g); Protein 22g; Phosphorus 265mg.*

Crab Imperial

PREP TIME: ABOUT 15 MIN	COOK TIME: 30 MIN	SERVINGS: 6	SERVING SIZE: 3 OUNCES (1 CUSTARD CUP)

INGREDIENTS

1 pound canned crabmeat, rinsed, drained, and flaked

1 egg white plus 2 tablespoons water, slightly beaten

½ cup low-fat mayonnaise

2 tablespoons fat-free milk

2 teaspoons capers, rinsed and drained

¼ cup finely chopped fresh dill

⅛ teaspoon freshly ground black pepper

Nonstick cooking spray

4 tablespoons Homemade Seasoned Bread Crumbs (see Chapter 14), divided

¼ cup chopped fresh parsley

DIRECTIONS

1 Preheat the oven to 350 degrees.

2 In a medium bowl, combine the crabmeat, egg, mayonnaise, milk, capers, dill, and pepper. Stir until well blended.

3 Coat 6 custard cups with nonstick cooking spray, and sprinkle 2 tablespoons of bread crumbs over the bottom of each. Divide the crab mixture evenly into the cups. Sprinkle the tops with the remaining 2 tablespoons of bread crumbs, and bake for 25–30 minutes at 350 degrees.

4 Remove from the oven, and garnish with the chopped parsley before serving.

TIP: This dish works great as a light party luncheon entree or as an appetizer for dinner.

PER SERVING: Choices/Exchanges ½ Carbohydrate, 1 Lean Protein; Calories 70 (from Fat 20); Fat 2g (Saturated 0.4g, Trans 0.0g); Cholesterol 45mg; Sodium 470mg; Potassium 240mg; Total Carbohydrate 6g (Dietary Fiber 0g, Sugars 1g); Protein 8g; Phosphorus 160mg.

Flounder Parmesan

INGREDIENTS

1 tablespoon extra-virgin olive oil

Four 4-ounce flounder filets

1 cup Marinara Sauce (see recipe, Chapter 6)

¼ cup freshly grated Parmigiano-Reggiano cheese

4 ounces skim milk mozzarella

DIRECTIONS

1 Preheat the oven to 375 degrees. Grease a baking dish with the olive oil, and place the fish filets on the dish.

2 Pour the Marina Sauce over the fish. Top with the Parmigiano-Reggiano Cheese and mozzarella. Bake for 12–15 minutes, or until the fish is cooked through and the mozzarella is bubbly. Transfer to a platter, and serve.

PER SERVING: *Choices/Exchanges 1 Nonstarchy Vegetable, 4 Lean Protein, 1 Fat; Calories 250 (from Fat 100); Fat 11g (Saturated 4.7g, Trans 0.0g); Cholesterol 85mg; Sodium 310mg; Potassium 530mg; Total Carbohydrate 6g (Dietary Fiber 2g, Sugars 3g); Protein 31g; Phosphorus 450mg.*

Grilled Salmon with Dill Sauce

PREP TIME: ABOUT 10 MIN	COOK TIME: 15 MIN	SERVINGS: 8	SERVING SIZE: 3–4 OUNCES SALMON WITH 2 TABLESPOONS SAUCE

INGREDIENTS

1 cup plain fat-free Greek yogurt

2 teaspoons minced fresh dill

¼ cup chopped scallions or onion

1 teaspoon capers

2 teaspoons minced fresh parsley

1 teaspoon minced fresh chives

Nonstick cooking spray

2 pounds salmon steaks

1 tablespoon extra-virgin olive oil

DIRECTIONS

1 In a small bowl, combine the yogurt, dill, scallions or onion, capers, parsley, and chives; set aside.

2 Spray the racks of your grill with nonstick cooking spray.

3 Brush the salmon steaks with olive oil, and grill them over medium–hot coals for 4 minutes per side, or just until the salmon flakes with a fork.

4 Transfer the salmon to a platter, and serve with the dill sauce on the side.

PER SERVING: *Choices/Exchanges 4 Lean Protein, ½ Fat; Calories 200 (from Fat 90); Fat 10g (Saturated 2.1g, Trans 0.0g); Cholesterol 65mg; Sodium 95mg; Potassium 450mg; Total Carbohydrate 1g (Dietary Fiber 0g, Sugars 1g); Protein 25g; Phosphorus 330mg.*

Grilled Scallop Kabobs

PREP TIME: ABOUT 15 MIN	COOK TIME: 20 MIN PLUS 30 MIN MARINADE	SERVINGS: 6	SERVING SIZE: 1 KABOB

INGREDIENTS

15 ounces pineapple chunks, packed in their own juice, undrained

¼ cup dry white wine

¼ cup light soy sauce

2 tablespoons minced fresh parsley

4 garlic cloves, minced

⅛ teaspoon freshly ground black pepper

1 pound scallops

18 large cherry tomatoes

1 large green bell pepper, cut into 1-inch squares

18 medium mushroom caps

DIRECTIONS

1 Drain the pineapple, reserving the juice. In a shallow baking dish, combine the pineapple juice, wine, soy sauce, parsley, garlic, and pepper. Mix well.

2 Add the pineapple, scallops, tomatoes, green pepper, and mushrooms to the marinade. Marinate 30 minutes at room temperature, stirring occasionally.

3 Alternate pineapple, scallops, and vegetables on metal or wooden skewers (remember to soak wooden skewers in water before using).

4 Grill the kabobs over medium-hot coals about 4–5 inches from the heat, turning frequently, for 5–7 minutes.

PER SERVING: *Choices/Exchanges ½ Fruit, 1 Nonstarchy Vegetable, 1 Lean Protein; Calories 120 (from Fat 10); Fat 1g (Saturated 0.2g, Trans 0.0g); Cholesterol 20mg; Sodium 260mg; Potassium 530mg; Total Carbohydrate 16g (Dietary Fiber 2g, Sugars 10g); Protein 13g; Phosphorus 270mg.*

Grilled Rosemary Swordfish

PREP TIME: ABOUT 5 MIN	COOK TIME: 15 MIN PLUS 30 MIN MARINADE	SERVINGS: 4	SERVING SIZE: 3 OUNCES

INGREDIENTS

2 scallions, thinly sliced

2 tablespoons extra-virgin olive oil

2 tablespoons white wine vinegar

1 teaspoon fresh rosemary, finely chopped

4 swordfish steaks (1 pound total)

DIRECTIONS

1 In a small bowl, combine the scallions, olive oil, vinegar, and rosemary. Pour over the swordfish steaks. Let the steaks marinate for 30 minutes.

2 Remove the steaks from the marinade, and grill for 5–7 minutes per side, brushing with marinade. Transfer to a serving platter, and serve.

VARY IT! Try grilling fresh vegetables, chicken, or tuna with this marinade as well.

PER SERVING: *Choices/Exchanges 3 Lean Protein, 1 ½ Fat; Calories 200 (from Fat 100); Fat 11g (Saturated 2.2g, Trans 0.0g); Cholesterol 45mg; Sodium 105mg; Potassium 350mg; Total Carbohydrate 1g (Dietary Fiber 0g, Sugars 0g); Protein 22g; Phosphorus 300mg.*

Halibut Supreme

PREP TIME: ABOUT 10 MIN	COOK TIME: 25 MIN	SERVINGS: 6	SERVING SIZE: 3 OUNCES

INGREDIENTS

Nonstick cooking spray

1½ pound halibut steaks

1 cup sliced mushrooms

1 tablespoon extra-virgin olive oil

1 small onion, finely chopped

3 tablespoons white wine

¾ cup water

⅛ teaspoon freshly ground black pepper

¼ teaspoon salt

¼ cup toasted almond slivers

1 tablespoon chopped fresh parsley

DIRECTIONS

1 Preheat the oven to 325 degrees. Coat a 13-x-9-x-2-inch baking dish with cooking spray, and place the halibut steaks in a baking dish.

2 Add the remaining ingredients except the almonds and parsley, and bake at 325 degrees, basting frequently, for 25 minutes until the fish flakes easily with a fork.

3 Remove from the oven, and top the halibut steaks with the toasted almond slivers. Garnish with parsley.

TIP: Add a variety of vegetables such as broccoli florets and diced pepper to this recipe for extra nutrients and an easy meal in a pan.

PER SERVING: *Choices/Exchanges 4 Lean Protein; Calories 180 (from Fat 60); Fat 7g (Saturated 0.9g, Trans 0.0g); Cholesterol 35mg; Sodium 160mg; Potassium 610mg; Total Carbohydrate 3g (Dietary Fiber 1g, Sugars 1g); Protein 25g; Phosphorus 290mg.*

Lobster Fricassee

PREP TIME: ABOUT 5 MIN | COOK TIME: 20 MIN | SERVINGS: 4 | SERVING SIZE: ½ CUP

INGREDIENTS

2 cups shelled lobster meat

1 tablespoon extra-virgin olive oil

¾ pound mushrooms, sliced

1 small onion, minced

½ cup fat-free milk

¼ cup flour

¼ teaspoon paprika

¼ teaspoon salt

⅛ teaspoon freshly ground black pepper

2 cups cooked whole-wheat pasta

¼ cup finely chopped parsley

DIRECTIONS

1 Cut the lobster meat into bite-size pieces. In a saucepan, heat the oil; add the mushrooms and onion, and sauté for 5–6 minutes.

2 In a small bowl, whisk the milk and flour, whisking quickly to eliminate any lumps. Pour the milk mixture into the mushroom mixture; mix thoroughly, and continue cooking for 3–5 minutes.

3 Add the lobster, paprika, salt, and pepper; continue cooking for 5–10 minutes until the lobster is heated through.

4 Spread the pasta onto a serving platter, spoon the lobster and sauce over the top, and garnish with parsley to serve.

PER SERVING: *Choices/Exchanges 2 Starch, 1 Nonstarchy Vegetable, 2 Lean Protein; Calories 260 (from Fat 50); Fat 6g (Saturated 0.9g, Trans 0.0g); Cholesterol 95mg; Sodium 480mg; Potassium 600mg; Total Carbohydrate 34g (Dietary Fiber 4g, Sugars 5g); Protein 21g; Phosphorus 330mg.*

Pan-Fried Scallops

PREP TIME: ABOUT 5 MIN	COOK TIME: 10 MIN	SERVINGS: 6	SERVING SIZE: 3–4 OUNCES

INGREDIENTS

½ cup Homemade Seasoned Bread Crumbs (see Chapter 14)

¼ teaspoon salt

⅛ teaspoon freshly ground black pepper

1½ pounds scallops

¼ cup extra-virgin olive oil

¼ cup dry white wine

4 roasted red peppers, cut into strips

1 bunch fresh parsley, finely minced

DIRECTIONS

1 In a small bowl, combine the bread crumbs, salt, and pepper. Roll the scallops thoroughly in the bread crumb mixture.

2 In a large skillet, heat the olive oil over medium high heat, and sauté the scallops quickly for 2–3 minutes until lightly browned.

3 Place the cooked scallops on top of the roasted red pepper strips on a serving dish.

4 Add the white wine to the remaining olive oil in the pan. Bring to a slow boil. Remove from the heat, and pour over the scallops. Top with parsley, and serve.

TIP: Be sure to use dry (preservative-free) scallops to get a nice brown seared finish.

PER SERVING: *Choices/Exchanges ½ Carbohydrate, 2 Lean Protein, 1½ Fat; Calories 200 (from Fat 90); Fat 10g (Saturated 1.5g, Trans 0.0g); Cholesterol 30mg; Sodium 420mg; Potassium 380mg; Total Carbohydrate 11g (Dietary Fiber 1g, Sugars 3g); Protein 16g; Phosphorus 335mg.*

Poached Red Snapper

PREP TIME: ABOUT 5 MIN	COOK TIME: 25 MIN	SERVINGS: 4	SERVING SIZE: 4 OUNCES

INGREDIENTS

1 cup dry white wine

1 medium lemon, sliced

6 parsley sprigs, plus additional for garnish

5 peppercorns

5 scallions, sliced

2 bay leaves

¼ teaspoon salt

1 cup water

1 red snapper (about 1½–2 pounds), cleaned and scaled with head and tail left on

1 lemon, sliced

DIRECTIONS

1 In a fish poacher or very large skillet, combine the wine, lemon slices, 6 parsley sprigs, peppercorns, scallions, bay leaves, salt, and water. Bring the mixture to a boil; add the snapper.

2 Cover the pan, lower the heat, and simmer the red snapper for 15–20 minutes until the fish flakes easily with a fork.

3 Carefully lift out the snapper, and transfer to a platter. Garnish with lemon slices and parsley.

VARY IT! Any fish could be prepared this way.

PER SERVING: *Choice/Exchanges 3 Lean Protein; Calories 120 (from Fat 15); Fat 1.5g (Saturated 0.0g, Trans 0.0g); Cholesterol 40mg; Sodium 95mg; Potassium 470mg; Total Carbohydrate 1g (Dietary Fiber 0g, Sugars 0g); Protein 22g; Phosphorus 220mg.*

Sea Bass with Ginger Sauce

PREP TIME: ABOUT 5 MIN	COOK TIME: 15 MIN	SERVINGS: 2	SERVING SIZE: 3–4 OUNCES

INGREDIENTS

Two 4-ounce sea bass filets

1 tablespoon extra-virgin olive oil

2 tablespoons minced fresh ginger

2 garlic cloves, minced

⅓ cup minced scallions

4 teaspoons chopped cilantro

1 tablespoon light soy sauce

DIRECTIONS

1 In a medium steamer, add water and bring to a boil. Arrange the filets on the steamer rack. Cover, and steam for 6–8 minutes.

2 Meanwhile, in a small skillet, heat the oil over medium-high heat. Add the ginger and garlic, and sauté for 2–3 minutes.

3 Transfer the steamed filets to a platter. Pour the ginger oil over the filets, and top with scallions, cilantro, and soy sauce.

PER SERVING: *Choices/Exchanges 3 Lean Protein, 1 Fat; Calories 190 (from Fat 80); Fat 9g (Saturated 1.5g, Trans 0.0g); Cholesterol 45mg; Sodium 360mg; Potassium 390mg; Total Carbohydrate 4g (Dietary Fiber 1g, Sugars 1g); Protein 22g; Phosphorus 240mg.*

Shrimp Creole

PREP TIME: ABOUT 5 MIN	COOK TIME: 20 MIN	SERVINGS: 4	SERVING SIZE: 2–3 OUNCES SHRIMP PLUS ½ CUP VEGETABLES

INGREDIENTS

One 8-ounce can no-salt-added fire-roasted tomatoes

½ cup sliced mushrooms

¼ cup dry white wine

½ cup chopped onion

2 garlic cloves, minced

1 cup chopped green bell pepper

1 cup chopped celery

2 bay leaves

¼ teaspoon cayenne pepper

1 pound shrimp, shelled and deveined

DIRECTIONS

1 In a large skillet, combine the tomatoes, mushrooms, wine, onion, garlic, green pepper, celery, bay leaves, and cayenne pepper. Bring to a boil; cover, reduce the heat, and let simmer for 10–15 minutes.

2 Add the shrimp to the tomato sauce, and cook uncovered for 3–5 minutes until the shrimp are bright pink.

3 Discard the bay leaves, and serve on a platter.

VARY IT! This creole sauce is really versatile; you can add chicken cubes, lobster chunks, mussels, or clams instead of shrimp.

TIP: If possible, use fresh (never frozen) shrimp or shrimp that are free of preservatives — for example, shrimp that have not been treated with salt or sodium tripolyphosphate (STPP).

PER SERVING: *Choices/Exchanges 2 Nonstarchy Vegetable, 2 Lean Protein; Calories 100 (from Fat 0); Fat 0g (Saturated 0.1g, Trans 0.0g); Cholesterol 120mg; Sodium 120mg; Potassium 490mg; Total Carbohydrate 8g (Dietary Fiber 2g, Sugars 4g); Protein 17g; Phosphorus 195mg.*

3

Whipping Up Sides and Supporting Dishes

Get creative with light, tasty appetizers for any occasion.

Enjoy the bright flavors of inspired salads and homemade dressings.

Dish out exciting vegetable sides that everyone will love.

Choose nutrient-rich rice and potato side dishes.

Warm up with unforgettable diabetes-friendly breads and muffins.

Bring joy to your meals with delightful desserts.

Chapter **10**

Appetizers

RECIPES IN THIS CHAPTER

When you think of appetizers, what comes to mind? Holidays and parties? Family time? A house full of friends and laughter? Eating healthy doesn't mean you have to miss out on the fun! This chapter is full of exciting, tasty little bites and rich, flavorful dips that are sure to wow your friends and family at any event. Whether you're hosting a formal party, bringing a dish to a friend's potluck, or just making your kids an after-school snack, you'll find a recipe to suit your needs. These appetizers taste decadent but won't disrupt your healthy eating efforts. Plus, they're quick and simple to prepare, which makes entertaining a snap.

Appetizers aren't just for special occasions; don't be afraid to work these delicious recipes into your everyday meal plan. Appetizers make great snacks and, if you choose the recipe wisely, they can actually be a good opportunity to add more servings of healthy foods into your day. For example, if your diabetes meal plan includes a snack, try a serving of one of the plant-based appetizers in this chapter, such as the Cucumber Pâté, Guacamole, or Hummus with some veggie sticks. Appetizer recipes can also be good additions to healthy meals. Try pairing a serving of the Baked Scallops, Broiled Shrimp with Garlic, or Chicken Kabobs with a salad or veggies for a light dinner. Get creative with these diabetes-friendly apps!

Baked Scallops

PREP TIME: ABOUT 5 MIN PLUS CHILLING TIME	COOK TIME: 10 MIN	SERVINGS: 4	SERVING SIZE: 3 OUNCES

INGREDIENTS

12 ounces fresh bay or dry sea scallops

1½ teaspoons salt-free pickling spices

½ cup cider vinegar

¼ cup water

1 tablespoon finely chopped onion

1 red bell pepper, cut into thin strips

1 head butter lettuce, rinsed and dried

⅓ cup sesame seeds, toasted

DIRECTIONS

1 Preheat the oven to 350 degrees. Wash the scallops in cool water, and cut any scallops that are too big in half.

2 Spread the scallops out in a large baking dish (be careful not to overlap them). In a small bowl, combine the spices, cider vinegar, water, onion, and pepper; pour the mixture over the scallops. Season with salt, if desired.

3 Cover the baking dish and bake for 7 minutes. Remove from the oven, and allow the scallops to chill in the refrigerator (leave them in the cooking liquid/vegetable mixture).

4 Just before serving, place the lettuce leaves on individual plates or a platter, and place the scallops and vegetables over the top. Sprinkle with sesame seeds before serving.

TIP: If possible use fresh (never frozen) scallops, or scallops that are free of preservatives — for example, scallops that have not been treated with salt or sodium tripolyphosphate (STPP). Spear these scallops with fancy toothpicks or serve them on a bed of butter lettuce as a prelude to a pasta dish. Remember not to overcook scallops; they'll become chewy instead of tender.

PER SERVING: *Choices/Exchanges ½ Carbohydrate, 2 Lean Protein, ½ Fat; Calories 150 (from Fat 50); Fat 6g (Saturated 0.9g, Trans 0.0g); Cholesterol 20mg; Sodium 150mg; Potassium 430mg; Total Carbohydrate 10g (Dietary Fiber 3g, Sugars 2g); Protein 14g; Phosphorus 325mg.*

Broiled Shrimp with Garlic

PREP TIME: ABOUT 5 MIN	COOK TIME: 10 MIN	SERVINGS: 12	SERVING SIZE: 2½ OUNCES

INGREDIENTS

2 pounds large shrimp, unshelled

⅓ cup extra-virgin olive oil

1 tablespoon lemon juice

¼ cup chopped scallions

1 tablespoon chopped garlic

2 teaspoons freshly ground black pepper

1 large lemon, sliced

4 tablespoons chopped fresh parsley

DIRECTIONS

1 Set the oven to broil. Shell the uncooked shrimp, but do not remove the tails. With a small knife, split the shrimp down the back, and remove the vein. Wash the shrimp with cool water, and pat dry with paper towels.

2 In a medium skillet, over medium heat, heat the olive oil. Add the lemon juice, scallions, garlic, and pepper. Heat the mixture for 3 minutes. Set aside.

3 In a baking dish, arrange the shrimp and pour the olive oil mixture over the shrimp. Broil the shrimp 4–5 inches from the heat for 2 minutes per side, just until the shrimp turns bright pink. Transfer the shrimp to a platter and garnish with lemon slices and parsley. Pour the juices from the pan over the shrimp.

TIP: If possible use fresh (never frozen) shrimp, or shrimp that are free of preservatives — for example, shrimp that have not been treated with salt or sodium tripolyphosphate (STPP). You can prepare this fast appetizer as guests are walking in, or serve it as a main course over rice. Make sure you buy 2 pounds of unshelled shrimp.

PER SERVING: Choices/Exchanges 2 Lean Protein, ½ Fat; Calories 100 (from Fat 50); Fat 6g (Saturated 0.9g, Trans 0.0g); Cholesterol 80mg; Sodium 50mg; Potassium 135mg; Total Carbohydrate 1g (Dietary Fiber 0g, Sugars 0g); Protein 10g; Phosphorus 105mg.

Cheesy Tortilla Wedges

PREP TIME: ABOUT 5 MIN	COOK TIME: 10MIN	SERVINGS: 12	SERVING SIZE: 3 WEDGES

INGREDIENTS

6 large corn tortillas (8 inches in diameter)

1 cup shredded fat-free cheddar cheese

3 tablespoons shredded reduced-fat Monterey Jack cheese

1 cup black beans, cooked, slightly mashed

½ cup green chilies

½ cup sliced pitted black olives

DIRECTIONS

1 Preheat the oven to 400 degrees. Place the tortillas on cookie sheets, and bake 5–7 minutes or until the edges start to curl.

2 Turn the tortillas over; top with the two cheeses, beans, chilies, and olives, spreading to the edge. Bake an additional 3 minutes or until the cheese melts.

3 Cut each tortilla into 6 wedges and arrange on a platter. Top with Guacamole (optional; see recipe later in this chapter), and serve.

PER SERVING: *Exchanges 1 Starch, ½ Fat; Calories 90 (from Fat 15); Fat 1.5g (Saturated 0.4g, Trans 0.0g); Cholesterol 2mg; Sodium 180mg; Potassium 125mg; Total Carbohydrate 14g (Dietary Fiber 3g, Sugars 1g); Protein 6g; Phosphorus 145mg.*

Chicken Kabobs

PREP TIME: ABOUT 5 MIN PLUS MARINATING TIME	COOK TIME: 20 MIN	SERVINGS: 6	SERVING SIZE: 2 SKEWERS

INGREDIENTS

1 pound boneless, skinless chicken breast

3 tablespoons light soy sauce

One 1-inch cube of fresh ginger root, finely chopped

3 tablespoons extra-virgin olive oil

3 tablespoons dry vermouth

1 large clove garlic, finely chopped

12 watercress sprigs

2 large lemons, cut into wedges

DIRECTIONS

1 Cut the chicken into 1-inch cubes and place in a shallow bowl.

2 In a small bowl, combine the soy sauce, ginger root, oil, vermouth, and garlic and pour over the chicken. Cover the chicken, and let marinate for at least 1 hour (or overnight).

3 Thread the chicken onto 12 metal or wooden skewers (remember to soak wooden skewers in water before using). Grill or broil 6 inches from the heat source for 8 minutes, turning frequently.

4 Arrange the skewers on a platter and garnish with the watercress and lemon wedges. Serve hot with additional soy sauce, if desired.

TIP: Serve these kabobs in the summer with roasted corn and squash.

PER SERVING: *Choices/Exchanges 2 Lean Protein; Calories 110 (from Fat 30); Fat 3.5g (Saturated 0.8g, Trans 0.0g); Cholesterol 45mg; Sodium 110mg; Potassium 170mg; Total Carbohydrate 2g (Dietary Fiber 0g, Sugars 1g); Protein 16g; Phosphorus 125mg.*

Chilled Shrimp

PREP TIME: ABOUT 5 MIN PLUS MARINATING TIME	COOK TIME: 5 MIN	SERVINGS: 20	SERVING SIZE: ½ CUP

INGREDIENTS

5 pounds jumbo shrimp, unshelled

¼ cup plus 2 tablespoons extra-virgin olive oil, divided

4 medium lemons, thinly sliced

3 tablespoons minced garlic

3 medium red onions, thinly sliced

½ cup minced parsley

Parsley sprigs (for garnish)

DIRECTIONS

1 Preheat the oven to 400 degrees. Peel, and devein shrimp, leaving the tails intact.

2 Arrange the shrimp on a baking sheet and brush with 2 tablespoons of the olive oil. Bake the shrimp for 3 minutes or until they turn bright pink.

3 Place the lemon slices in a large bowl. Add the remaining ¼ cup of olive oil, garlic, onions, and minced parsley. Add the shrimp and toss vigorously to coat. Cover, and let marinate, refrigerated, for 6–8 hours.

4 Just before serving, arrange the shrimp on a serving platter. Garnish with parsley sprigs and some of the red onions and lemons from the bowl.

TIP: If possible use fresh (never frozen) shrimp, or shrimp that are free of preservatives — for example, shrimp that have not been treated with salt or sodium tripolyphosphate (STPP).

PER SERVING: *Choices/Exchanges 2 Lean Protein; Calories 90 (from Fat 20); Fat 2.5g (Saturated 0.3g, Trans 0.0g); Cholesterol 120mg; Sodium 75mg; Potassium 220mg; Total Carbohydrate 3g (Dietary Fiber 0g, Sugars 1g); Protein 16g; Phosphorus 160mg.*

Crab-Filled Mushrooms

| PREP TIME: ABOUT 5 MIN | COOK TIME: 25 MIN | SERVINGS: 10 | SERVING SIZE: 2 MUSHROOM CAPS |

INGREDIENTS

20 large fresh mushroom caps

6 ounces canned crabmeat, rinsed, drained, and flaked

½ cup crushed whole-wheat crackers

2 tablespoons chopped fresh parsley

2 tablespoons finely chopped green onion

⅛ teaspoon freshly ground black pepper

¼ cup chopped pimiento

3 tablespoons extra-virgin olive oil

10 tablespoons wheat germ

DIRECTIONS

1 Preheat the oven to 350 degrees. Clean the mushrooms by dusting off any dirt on the cap with a mushroom brush or paper towel; remove the stems.

2 In a small mixing bowl, combine the crabmeat, crackers, parsley, onion, and pepper.

3 Place the mushroom caps in a 13-x-9-x-2-inch baking dish, crown side down. Stuff some of the crabmeat filling into each cap. Place a little pimiento on top of the filling.

4 Drizzle the olive oil over the caps and sprinkle each cap with ½ tablespoon wheat germ. Bake for 15–17 minutes. Transfer to a serving platter, and serve hot.

VARY IT! This is a very versatile filling you can also stuff into cherry tomatoes, zucchini, or yellow squash "boats" (cut 2-inch pieces of squash and scoop out the middles).

PER SERVING: *Choices/Exchanges ½ Starch, 1 Fat; Calories 100 (from Fat 50); Fat 6g (Saturated 0.9g, Trans 0.0g); Cholesterol 10mg; Sodium 95mg; Potassium 280mg; Total Carbohydrate 8g (Dietary Fiber 2g, Sugars 2g); Protein 5g; Phosphorus 160mg.*

Cucumber Pâté

PREP TIME: ABOUT 10 MIN PLUS CHILLING TIME	COOK TIME: 20 MIN	SERVINGS: 12	SERVING SIZE: ½ CUP

INGREDIENTS

1 large cucumber, peeled, seeded, and quartered

1 small green bell pepper, seeded and quartered

3 stalks celery, quartered

1 medium onion, quartered

1 cup low-fat cottage cheese

½ cup plain nonfat Greek yogurt

1 package unflavored gelatin

¼ cup boiling water

¼ cup cold water

DIRECTIONS

1 Spray a 5-cup mold or a 1½-quart mixing bowl with nonstick cooking spray.

2 In a food processor, coarsely chop the cucumber, green pepper, celery, and onion. Remove the vegetables from the food processor and set aside.

3 In a food processor, combine the cottage cheese and yogurt, and blend until smooth.

4 In a medium bowl, dissolve the gelatin in the boiling water; slowly stir in the cold water. Add the chopped vegetables and cottage cheese mixture, and mix thoroughly.

5 Pour the mixture into the prepared mold and refrigerate overnight or until firm. To serve, carefully invert the mold onto a serving plate, and remove the mold. Surround the pâté with assorted crackers, and serve.

TIP: You might want to make this tasty pâté the day before your party, so it can solidify in the refrigerator overnight.

PER SERVING: *Choices/Exchanges 1 Nonstarchy Vegetable; Calories 30 (from Fat 0); Fat 0g (Saturated 0.2g, Trans 0.0g); Cholesterol 0mg; Sodium 95mg; Potassium 120mg; Total Carbohydrate 3g (Dietary Fiber 1g, Sugars 2g); Protein 4g; Phosphorus 50mg.*

Fresh Dill Dip

PREP TIME: ABOUT 5 MIN PLUS CHILLING TIME	COOK TIME: 5 MIN	SERVINGS: 6	SERVING SIZE: 2 TABLESPOONS

INGREDIENTS

1 cup plain fat-free yogurt

¼ teaspoon salt

¼ teaspoon freshly ground black pepper

¼ cup minced parsley

2 tablespoons finely chopped fresh chives

1 tablespoon finely chopped fresh dill

1 tablespoon apple cider vinegar

DIRECTIONS

1 In a small bowl, combine all the ingredients. Chill for 2–4 hours. Serve with fresh cut vegetables.

PER SERVING: *Choices/Exchanges Free Food; Calories 20 (from Fat 0); Fat 0g (Saturated 0.0g, Trans 0.0g); Cholesterol 0mg; Sodium 125mg; Potassium 105mg; Total Carbohydrate 3g (Dietary Fiber 0g, Sugars 3g); Protein 2g; Phosphorus 60mg.*

Gruyere Apple Spread

PREP TIME: ABOUT 5 MIN PLUS CHILLING TIME	COOK TIME: 5 MIN	SERVINGS: 20	SERVING SIZE: 1 TABLESPOON

INGREDIENTS

4 ounces fat-free cream cheese, softened

½ cup low-fat cottage cheese

4 ounces Gruyere cheese

¼ teaspoon dry mustard

⅛ teaspoon freshly ground black pepper

½ cup shredded apple (unpeeled)

2 tablespoons finely chopped pecans

2 teaspoons minced fresh chives

DIRECTIONS

1 Place the cheeses in a food processor, and blend until smooth. Add the mustard and pepper, and blend for 30 seconds.

2 Transfer the mixture to a serving bowl, and fold in the apple and pecans. Sprinkle the dip with chives.

3 Cover, and refrigerate the mixture for 1–2 hours. Serve chilled with crackers, or stuff into celery stalks.

PER SERVING: *Choices/Exchanges ½ Fat; Calories 40 (from Fat 20); Fat 2.5g (Saturated 1.2g, Trans 0.0g); Cholesterol 5mg; Sodium 100mg; Potassium 30mg; Total Carbohydrate 1g (Dietary Fiber 0g, Sugars 1g); Protein 3g; Phosphorus 75mg.*

Guacamole

INGREDIENTS

2 large (8½-ounce) ripe avocados, peeled, pits removed, and mashed

½ cup chopped onion

2 medium jalapeño peppers, seeded and chopped

2 tablespoons minced fresh parsley

2 tablespoons fresh lime juice

⅛ teaspoon freshly ground black pepper

2 medium tomatoes, finely chopped

1 medium garlic clove, minced

1 tablespoon extra-virgin olive oil

½ teaspoon salt

DIRECTIONS

1 In a large mixing bowl, combine all ingredients, blending well.

TIP: There's a secret to selecting perfectly ripe avocados: Look for slightly blackened ones that give just a little when you press on their skins.

PER SERVING: *Choices/Exchanges 1 Nonstarchy Vegetable, 1½ Fat; Calories 100 (from Fat 70); Fat 8g (Saturated 1.2g, Trans 0.0g); Cholesterol 0mg; Sodium 150mg; Potassium 360mg; Total Carbohydrate 8g (Dietary Fiber 4g, Sugars 2g); Protein 2g; Phosphorus 40mg.*

Hot Artichoke Dip

PREP TIME: ABOUT 5 MIN	COOK TIME: 20 MIN	SERVINGS: 12	SERVING SIZE: 2 TABLESPOONS

INGREDIENTS

Two 9-ounce packages frozen artichoke hearts, thawed

2 cloves garlic

2 tablespoons extra-virgin olive oil

⅓ cup fresh lemon juice

¼ teaspoon hot pepper sauce

¼ cup grated fresh Parmigiano-Reggiano cheese

1½ cups dried whole-wheat bread crumbs

¼ cup finely chopped basil

DIRECTIONS

1 Preheat the oven to 350 degrees.

2 In a blender or food processor, combine the artichoke hearts, garlic, olive oil, lemon juice, and hot pepper sauce and puree for 30 seconds.

3 Pour the puree into a large bowl; stir in the cheese, bread crumbs, and basil. Transfer the mixture to a 1-quart baking dish.

4 Cover the dip, and bake at 350 degrees for 15 minutes or until lightly golden brown. Serve warm with crackers or bread.

PER SERVING: *Choices/Exchanges ½ Carbohydrate; Calories 45 (from Fat 15); Fat 1.5g (Saturated 0.4g, Trans 0.0g); Cholesterol 0mg; Sodium 25mg; Potassium 70mg; Total Carbohydrate 6g (Dietary Fiber 2g, Sugars 1g); Protein 2g, Phosphorus 30mg.*

Hummus

PREP TIME: ABOUT 5 MIN	COOK TIME: 5 MIN	SERVINGS: 12	SERVING SIZE: 2 TABLESPOONS

INGREDIENTS

One 15-ounce can chickpeas, drained (reserve a little liquid)

3 cloves garlic

Juice of 1 lemon

Juice of 1 lime

1 teaspoon extra-virgin olive oil

1 teaspoon ground cumin

DIRECTIONS

1 In a blender or food processor, combine all the ingredients until smooth, adding chickpea liquid or water if necessary to blend, and create a creamy texture. Refrigerate until ready to serve. Serve with crunchy vegetables, crackers, or pita bread.

PER SERVING: *Choices/Exchanges ½ Starch; Calories 40 (from Fat 10); Fat 1.0g (Saturated 0.1g, Trans 0.0g); Cholesterol 0mg; Sodium 40mg; Potassium 70mg; Total Carbohydrate 6g (Dietary Fiber 2g, Sugars 1g); Protein 2g; Phosphorus 35mg.*

Creamy Cheese Dip

PREP TIME: ABOUT 5 MIN	COOK TIME: 5 MIN	SERVINGS: 40	SERVING SIZE: 1 TABLESPOON

INGREDIENTS

1 cup plain fat-free yogurt, strained overnight in cheesecloth over a bowl set in the refrigerator

1 cup fat-free ricotta cheese

1 cup low-fat cottage cheese

DIRECTIONS

1 Combine all the ingredients in a food processor; process until smooth. Place in a covered container, and refrigerate until ready to use (this cream cheese can be refrigerated for up to 1 week).

PER SERVING: *Choices/Exchanges Free Food; Calories 10 (from Fat 0); Fat 0g (Saturated 0.0g, Trans 0.0g); Cholesterol 0mg; Sodium 30mg; Potassium 20mg; Total Carbohydrate 1g (Dietary Fiber 0g, Sugars 1g); Protein 2g; Phosphorus 25mg.*

Monterey Jack Cheese Quiche Squares

PREP TIME: ABOUT 10 MIN	COOK TIME: 15 MIN	SERVINGS: 12	SERVING SIZE: 1 SQUARE

INGREDIENTS

4 egg whites

1 cup plus 2 tablespoons low-fat cottage cheese

¼ cup plus 2 tablespoons flour

¾ teaspoon baking powder

1 cup shredded reduced-fat Monterey Jack cheese

½ cup diced green chilies

1 red bell pepper, diced

1 cup lentils, cooked

1 tablespoon extra-virgin olive oil

Parsley sprigs

DIRECTIONS

1 Preheat the oven to 350 degrees.

2 In a medium bowl, beat the egg whites and cottage cheese for 2 minutes, until smooth.

3 Add the flour and baking powder, and beat until smooth. Stir in the cheese, green chilies, red pepper, and lentils.

4 Coat a 9-inch-square pan with the olive oil, and pour in the egg mixture. Bake for 30–35 minutes, until firm.

5 Remove the quiche from the oven, and allow to cool for 10 minutes (it will be easier to cut). Cut into 12 squares and transfer to a platter, garnish with parsley sprigs, and serve.

PER SERVING: *Choices/Exchanges ½ Starch, 1 Lean Protein; Calories 100 (from Fat 30); Fat 3.5g (Saturated 1.5g, Trans 0.0g); Cholesterol 10mg; Sodium 210mg; Potassium 170mg; Total Carbohydrate 9g (Dietary Fiber 2g, Sugars 2g); Protein 8g; Phosphorus 140mg.*

Chapter **11**

Salads and Dressings

RECIPES IN THIS CHAPTER

B right salads with tasty dressings are a great opportunity for people with diabetes to include fresh, healthy ingredients in their meal plan. Fitting enough servings of fruits and veggies into your diet can be challenging for everyone, not just people with diabetes. But salads with homemade dressings are a quick and easy way to get the nutrients your body craves. If you think salads are boring, think again. This chapter includes both vegetable-based salad recipes and heartier potato-, pasta-, and grain-based salads — all of which are diabetes friendly. The variety of flavors, textures, and delicious proteins in these recipes will leave you feeling satisfied and loving salads.

Don't underestimate the power of a good dressing. The right dressing can turn even a simple salad into a meal to remember. But store-bought dressings are often full of fat and sodium. The dressing recipes in this chapter feature fresh herbs, spices, and vegetables; healthy fats; and zingy citrus.

After you've tasted one of these healthy homemade dressings, you won't want to go back to store-bought condiments.

REMEMBER

Don't be afraid to think outside the box when it comes to salads and dressings. You can make a salad with any combination of vegetables, fruits, proteins, and even healthy whole grains. If you don't like one of the ingredients in a salad recipe, substitute it with another wholesome ingredient that fits with your meal plan. If you love one of the dressing recipes in this chapter, repurpose it, and use it as a marinade for protein or vegetables. The possibilities are endless!

Fiery Black Bean Salad

PREP TIME: ABOUT 10 MIN PLUS CHILLING TIME | SERVINGS: 8 | SERVING SIZE: 1 CUP

INGREDIENTS

3 cups cooked black beans

2 tomatoes, chopped

2 red bell peppers, finely chopped

1 cup yellow corn

3 garlic cloves, minced

1 jalapeño pepper, minced

¼ cup fresh lime juice

2 tablespoons red wine vinegar

1 tablespoon cumin

1 tablespoon extra-virgin olive oil

2 tablespoons freshly chopped cilantro (optional)

DIRECTIONS

1 Combine all ingredients in a bowl, and chill in the refrigerator for several hours to blend the flavors. Serve.

VARY IT! Use chickpeas instead of black beans if desired. Try adding grilled chicken or pork to this spicy salad.

TIP: Since this salad should be made ahead of time, it's perfect for entertaining.

PER SERVING: *Choices/Exchanges 1 Starch, 1 Nonstarchy Vegetable, 1 Lean Protein; Calories 140 (from Fat 20); Fat 2.5g (Saturated 0.4g, Trans 0.0g); Cholesterol 0mg; Sodium 5mg; Potassium 480mg; Total Carbohydrate 24g (Dietary Fiber 7g, Sugars 5g); Protein 7g; Phosphorus 130mg.*

Chinese Chicken Salad

PREP TIME: ABOUT 10 MIN PLUS CHILLING TIME | SERVINGS: 4 | SERVING SIZE: 6–8 OUNCES (2 TOMATOES EACH)

INGREDIENTS

2 cups cooked chicken, diced

1 cup finely chopped celery

1 cup shredded carrots

¼ cup crushed unsweetened pineapple, drained

2 tablespoons finely diced pimiento

Two 8-ounce cans water chestnuts, drained and chopped

2 scallions, chopped

⅓ cup low-fat mayonnaise

1 tablespoon light soy sauce

1 teaspoon lemon juice

8 large tomatoes, hollowed

DIRECTIONS

1 In a large bowl, combine the chicken, celery, carrots, pineapple, pimiento, water chestnuts, and scallions.

2 In a separate bowl, combine the mayonnaise, soy sauce, and lemon juice. Mix well. Add the dressing to the salad, and toss. Cover, and chill in the refrigerator for 2–3 hours.

3 For each serving, place a small scoop of chicken salad into a hollowed-out tomato.

VARY IT! Try stuffing the chicken salad into celery stalks or serve on bread.

PER SERVING: *Choices/Exchanges 6 Nonstarchy Vegetable, 2 Lean Protein, 1 Fat; Calories 280 (from Fat 60); Fat 7g (Saturated 1.7g, Trans 0.0g); Cholesterol 60mg; Sodium 460mg; Potassium 1220mg; Total Carbohydrate 30g (Dietary Fiber 8g, Sugars 14g); Protein 25g; Phosphorus 260mg.*

Couscous Salad

PREP TIME: ABOUT 10 MIN | SERVINGS: 6 | SERVING SIZE: ½ CUP

INGREDIENTS

1 cup whole-wheat couscous

2 cups boiling water

¼ cup finely chopped red or yellow bell pepper

¼ cup chopped carrots

¼ cup finely chopped celery

2 tablespoons minced Italian parsley

1 tablespoon extra-virgin olive oil

4 tablespoons rice vinegar

2 garlic cloves, minced

3 tablespoons finely minced scallions

¼ cup slivered almonds

¼ teaspoon freshly ground black pepper

DIRECTIONS

1 Place dry couscous in a heat-proof bowl. Pour boiling water over it, and let sit for 5–10 minutes until all the water is absorbed.

2 In a large bowl, combine the couscous, bell pepper, carrots, celery, and parsley together.

3 In a blender or food processor, combine the olive oil, vinegar, garlic, and scallions, and process for 1 minute. Pour over the couscous and vegetables, toss well, garnish with almonds, and season with the pepper. Serve.

PER SERVING: *Choices/Exchanges 1 ½ Starch, 1 Fat; Calories 160 (from Fat 45); Fat 5g (Saturated 0.5g, Trans 0.0g); Cholesterol 0mg; Sodium 10mg; Potassium 140mg; Total Carbohydrate 25g (Dietary Fiber 4g, Sugars 2g); Protein 5g; Phosphorus 80mg.*

Crab and Rice Salad

PREP TIME: ABOUT 10 MIN	COOK TIME: 45–50 MIN	SERVINGS: 4	SERVING SIZE: APPROXIMATELY 1 CUP

INGREDIENTS

1 cup uncooked brown rice

5 ounces cooked fresh crabmeat, flaked

1 large tomato, diced

One 1.8-ounce can sliced water chestnuts, drained

¼ cup chopped green bell pepper

3 tablespoons chopped fresh parsley

2 tablespoons minced red onion

½ cup plain fat-free yogurt

1½ tablespoons lemon juice

¼ teaspoon freshly ground black pepper

1 head butter lettuce, cored and quartered

1 large tomato, cut into wedges

DIRECTIONS

1 In a medium saucepan, boil 2½ cups of water. Slowly add the brown rice. Cover, and reduce the heat to low. Cook the rice for 45–50 minutes until tender. Do not continually stir the rice (this will cause it to become gummy). Just check it occasionally.

2 In a large salad bowl, combine all the ingredients except the lettuce and tomato wedges. Just before serving, line 4 plates with the lettuce, and spoon the salad on top of the lettuce. Garnish with the tomato wedges.

PER SERVING: *Choices/Exchanges 2½ Starch, 2 Nonstarchy Vegetable; Calories 250 (from Fat 20); Fat 2g (Saturated 0.4g, Trans 0.0g); Cholesterol 35mg; Sodium 180mg; Potassium 630mg; Total Carbohydrate 47g (Dietary Fiber 5g, Sugars 7g); Protein 14g; Phosphorus 300mg.*

Greek Island Potato Salad

PREP TIME: ABOUT 5 MIN	COOK TIME: 35 MIN	SERVINGS: 10	SERVING SIZE: ½ CUP

INGREDIENTS

⅓ cup extra-virgin olive oil

4 garlic cloves, minced

2 pounds red potatoes, cut into 1½-inch pieces (leave the skin on if you wish)

6 medium carrots, peeled, halved lengthwise, and cut into 1½-inch pieces

1 onion, chopped

16 ounces artichoke hearts packed in water, drained and cut in half

½ cup Kalamata olives, pitted and halved

¼ cup lemon juice

DIRECTIONS

1 In a large skillet, heat the olive oil. Add the garlic, and sauté for 30 seconds. Add the potatoes, carrots, and onion; cook over medium heat for 25–30 minutes until vegetables are just tender.

2 Add the artichoke hearts, and cook for 3–5 minutes more. Remove from the heat, and stir in the olives and lemon juice. Season with a dash of salt and pepper. Transfer to a serving bowl, and serve warm.

TIP: You can find Kalamata olives (Greek olives) at your supermarket or at a gourmet deli.

PER SERVING: *Choices/Exchanges 1 Starch, 2 Nonstarchy Vegetable, 1½ Fat; Calories 190 (from Fat 80); Fat 9g (Saturated 1.3g, Trans 0.0g); Cholesterol 0mg; Sodium 220mg; Potassium 620mg; Total Carbohydrate 24g (Dietary Fiber 4g, Sugars 4g); Protein 3g; Phosphorus 90mg.*

Haricot Verts, Walnut, and Feta Salad

PREP TIME: ABOUT 10 MIN PLUS CHILLING TIME	COOK TIME: 15 MIN	SERVINGS: 12	SERVING SIZE: ½ CUP

INGREDIENTS

½ cup walnuts, toasted

1½ pounds fresh haricot verts, trimmed and halved

½ cup cooked green lentils

1 medium red onion, sliced into rings

½ cup peeled, seeded, and diced cucumber

⅓ cup crumbled fat-free feta cheese

¼ cup extra-virgin olive oil

¼ cup white wine vinegar

¼ cup chopped fresh mint leaves

1 garlic clove, minced

DIRECTIONS

1 Place the walnuts in a small baking dish in a 350-degree oven for 5–10 minutes until lightly browned. Remove from the oven, and set aside.

2 Steam the haricot verts about 4–5 minutes, or until desired degree of crispness.

3 In a salad bowl, combine the haricot verts with the walnuts, lentils, red onion rings, cucumber, and feta cheese.

4 Combine all the dressing ingredients together, and toss with the vegetables. Chill in the refrigerator for 2–3 hours before serving.

PER SERVING: *Choices/Exchanges 2 Nonstarchy Vegetable, 1½ Fat; Calories 110 (from Fat 70); Fat 8g (Saturated 1.0g, Trans 0.0g); Cholesterol 0mg; Sodium 30mg; Potassium 160mg; Total Carbohydrate 8g (Dietary Fiber 3g, Sugars 2g); Protein 3g; Phosphorus 65mg.*

Italian Potato Salad

PREP TIME: ABOUT 10 MIN	COOK TIME: 25 MIN	SERVINGS: 8	SERVING SIZE: ½ CUP

INGREDIENTS

12 new red potatoes, 3–4 ounces each, washed and skins left on

3 celery stalks, chopped

1 red bell pepper, minced

¼ cup chopped scallions

2 tablespoons olive oil

1 tablespoon balsamic vinegar

½ tablespoon red vinegar

1 teaspoon chopped fresh parsley

⅛ teaspoon freshly ground black pepper

DIRECTIONS

1 Boil the potatoes for 20 minutes in a large pot of boiling water. Drain, and let cool for 30 minutes.

2 Cut the potatoes into large chunks, and toss the potatoes with the celery, bell pepper, and scallions.

3 In a medium bowl, combine the olive oil, balsamic vinegar, red vinegar, parsley, and pepper; pour the dressing over the potato salad. Serve at room temperature.

TIP: Leave the skins on the red potatoes for a rustic look.

PER SERVING: *Choices/Exchanges 2 Starch, ½ Fat; Calories 170 (from Fat 30); Fat 3.5g (Saturated 0.5g, Trans 0.0g); Cholesterol 0mg; Sodium 25mg; Potassium 650mg; Total Carbohydrate 31g (Dietary Fiber 4g, Sugars 3g); Protein 3g; Phosphorus 75mg.*

Lentil Salad

PREP TIME: ABOUT 10 MIN PLUS CHILLING TIME	COOK TIME: 45 MIN	SERVINGS: 8	SERVING SIZE: 1 CUP

INGREDIENTS

1 pound dried lentils, washed (rinse with cold water in a colander)

3 cups water

2 tablespoons extra-virgin olive oil

2 teaspoons cumin

1 teaspoon minced fresh oregano

3 tablespoons fresh lemon juice

¼ teaspoon freshly ground black pepper

2 large green bell peppers, cored, seeded, and diced

2 large red bell peppers, cored, seeded, and diced

3 stalks celery, diced

1 red onion, minced

DIRECTIONS

1 In a large saucepan over high heat, bring lentils and water to a boil. Reduce the heat to low, cover, and simmer for 35–45 minutes. Drain, and set aside.

2 In a large bowl, mix together the oil, cumin, oregano, lemon juice, and pepper until well blended. Add the lentils and the prepared vegetables. Cover, and chill in the refrigerator before serving.

TIP: The flavor of this filling salad improves with time, so you can leave the leftovers in the refrigerator for 2–3 days and serve it again!

PER SERVING: *Choices/Exchanges 2 Starch, 2 Nonstarchy Vegetable, 1 Lean Protein; Calories 250 (from Fat 40); Fat 4.5g (Saturated 0.6g, Trans 0.0g); Cholesterol 0mg; Sodium 25mg; Potassium 840mg; Total Carbohydrate 39g (Dietary Fiber 15g, Sugars 7g); Protein 15g; Phosphorus 310mg.*

Lobster Salad

PREP TIME: ABOUT 10 MIN	COOK TIME: 45 MIN	SERVINGS: 6	SERVING SIZE: ½ CUP

INGREDIENTS

2 pounds lobster in the shell or 1 pound lobster meat

¾ pound small red potatoes

½ cup light mayonnaise

3 tablespoons plain low-fat yogurt

1 tablespoon chopped tarragon

¼ cup chopped scallions

¼ teaspoon freshly ground black pepper

1 small head romaine lettuce, washed and leaves separated

DIRECTIONS

1 To prepare lobster in the shell, place the lobster in boiling water, and boil until the meat is tender, about 20 minutes. Cool the lobster, remove the meat from the shell, and cut into 1-inch cubes. Or buy lobster meat from the seafood department at the supermarket.

2 Wash, but do not peel, the potatoes. Boil the potatoes in water until just tender, about 15–20 minutes. Drain, cool, and quarter.

3 In a bowl, combine mayonnaise, yogurt, tarragon, scallions, and pepper for the dressing.

4 In a separate bowl, combine the lobster and potatoes.

5 Add the dressing to the lobster and potatoes, and mix well. To serve, line plates with lettuce. Spoon lobster salad over the lettuce.

PER SERVING: *Choices/Exchanges 1 Starch, 2 Lean Protein; Calories 160 (Calories from Fat 45); Total Fat 5g (Saturated Fat 0.6g, Trans 0.0g); Cholesterol 95mg; Sodium 460mg; Potassium 510mg; Total Carbohydrate 15g (Dietary Fiber 2g, Sugars 2g); Protein 14g; Phosphorus 170mg.*

Mediterranean Chicken Salad

PREP TIME: ABOUT 5 MIN PLUS CHILLING TIME | SERVINGS: 3 | SERVING SIZE: 1 CUP

INGREDIENTS

8 ounces boneless, skinless, cooked chicken breast

2 tablespoons extra-virgin olive oil

2 tablespoons balsamic vinegar

¼ teaspoon dried basil

2 small garlic cloves, minced

¼ teaspoon freshly ground black pepper

1 cup cooked green beans, cut into 2-inch pieces

1 cup cooked artichokes

¼ cup pine nuts, toasted

¼ cup sliced black olives

3 cherry tomatoes, halved

Tomato wedges (optional)

DIRECTIONS

1 Cut the cooked chicken into bite-sized chunks, and set aside.

2 In a medium bowl, whisk together the oil, vinegar, basil, garlic, and pepper. Add the chicken, and toss with the dressing.

3 Add the green beans, artichokes, pine nuts, olives, and cherry tomatoes; toss well. Chill in the refrigerator for several hours. Garnish the salad with tomato wedges, and serve.

VARY IT! Try adding crumbled fat-free feta cheese to this salad to give it more of a Greek flair.

PER SERVING: *Choices/Exchanges 3 Nonstarchy Vegetable, 3 Lean Protein, 3 Fat; Calories 350 (from Fat 190); Fat 21g (Saturated 2.8g, Trans 0.0g); Cholesterol 65mg; Sodium 180mg; Potassium 540mg; Total Carbohydrate 15g (Dietary Fiber 7g, Sugars 3g); Protein 28g; Phosphorus 300mg.*

Make-Ahead Apple, Carrot, and Cabbage Slaw

PREP TIME: ABOUT 10 MIN PLUS CHILLING TIME	SERVINGS: 6	SERVING SIZE: APPROXIMATELY 1 CUP

INGREDIENTS

4 cups shredded cabbage (green or purple, or a mixture)

2 cups shredded carrots

¾ cup sliced scallions

¾ cup unsweetened apple juice

⅔ cup cider vinegar

1½ teaspoons paprika

1 teaspoon mustard seeds

½ teaspoon garlic powder

½ teaspoon celery seeds

⅛ teaspoon freshly ground black pepper

1 tablespoon dry mustard

DIRECTIONS

1 In a large bowl, combine the cabbage, carrots, and scallions.

2 In a blender, combine the remaining ingredients. Pour over the cabbage mixture, and toss to coat. Refrigerate overnight, and serve chilled.

VARY IT! Grated red beets are a wonderful substitution for cabbage in this salad.

PER SERVING: *Choices/Exchanges 2 Nonstarchy Vegetable; Calories 60 (from Fat 10); Fat 1g (Saturated 0.1g, Trans 0.0g); Cholesterol 0mg; Sodium 35mg; Potassium 290mg; Total Carbohydrate 11g (Dietary Fiber 3g, Sugars 7g); Protein 2g; Phosphorus 45mg.*

Pasta Salad–Stuffed Tomatoes

PREP TIME: ABOUT 10 MIN PLUS CHILLING TIME	SERVINGS: 4	SERVING SIZE: ⅔ CUP STUFFING IN 1 TOMATO

INGREDIENTS:

1 cup uncooked whole-wheat fusilli

2 small carrots, sliced

2 scallions, chopped

¼ cup chopped pimiento

1 cup cooked kidney beans

½ cup sliced celery

¼ cup cooked peas

2 tablespoons chopped fresh parsley

¼ cup calorie-free, fat-free Italian salad dressing

2 tablespoons low-fat mayonnaise

¼ teaspoon dried marjoram

¼ teaspoon freshly ground black pepper

4 medium tomatoes

DIRECTIONS

1 Cook the fusilli in boiling water until cooked, about 7–8 minutes; drain.

2 In a large bowl, combine the macaroni with the remaining salad ingredients (except the tomatoes), and toss well. Cover, and chill in the refrigerator 1 hour or more.

3 With the stem end down, cut each tomato into 6 wedges, cutting to, but not through, the base of the tomato. Spread the wedges slightly apart, and spoon the pasta mixture into the tomatoes. Chill until ready to serve.

VARY IT! In Italy, tomatoes are also stuffed with rice and served while dining alfresco.

PER SERVING: *Choices/Exchanges 2 Starch, 2 Nonstarchy Vegetable; Calories 210 (from Fat 15); Fat 1.5g (Saturated 0.3g, Trans 0.0g); Cholesterol 0mg; Sodium 270mg; Potassium 820mg; Total Carbohydrate 43g (Dietary Fiber 9g, Sugars 8g); Protein 10g; Phosphorus 215mg.*

Shanghai Salad

INGREDIENTS

3 tablespoons canola oil

1 teaspoon grated fresh ginger

1 garlic clove, minced

8 ounces cooked lean flank steak, cut into 1-inch pieces

1½ cups fresh snow peas, trimmed

One 8-ounce can water chestnuts, drained and sliced

6 scallions, cut into 2-inch pieces

2 tablespoons dry sherry

1 tablespoon light soy sauce

4 cups romaine lettuce, shredded

DIRECTIONS

1 In a large skillet, heat the oil over medium–high heat. Sauté the ginger, and garlic for 1–2 minutes.

2 Add the remaining ingredients (except the lettuce) to the skillet, and stir until heated through.

3 Arrange the shredded lettuce on a platter, spoon the mixture over the bed of lettuce, and serve.

PER SERVING: *Choices/Exchanges 2 Nonstarchy Vegetable, 2 Lean Protein, 2½ Fat; Calories 260 (from Fat 140); Fat 15g (Saturated 2.5g, Trans 0.0g); Cholesterol 45mg; Sodium 190mg; Potassium 510mg; Total Carbohydrate 11g (Dietary Fiber 4g, Sugars 3g); Protein 18g; Phosphorus 175mg.*

Shrimp and Radicchio Salad

PREP TIME: ABOUT 10 MIN PLUS CHILLING TIME ·	SERVINGS: 4	SERVING SIZE: APPROXIMATELY 1/3 CUP SHRIMP AND MARINADE PLUS ½ CUP LETTUCE AND RADICCHIO

INGREDIENTS

¼ cup olive oil

2 tablespoons red wine vinegar

3 medium garlic cloves, minced

1 medium shallot, minced

2 teaspoons Dijon mustard

1 teaspoon prepared horseradish

¼ teaspoon freshly ground black pepper

½ pound fresh (never frozen) cooked bay shrimp

1 medium head Boston lettuce, shredded

1 medium head radicchio lettuce, shredded

DIRECTIONS

1 In a medium bowl, combine the olive oil, vinegar, garlic, shallots, mustard, horseradish, and pepper. Add the shrimp, and toss well. Chill in the refrigerator for 30 minutes.

2 Just before serving, combine the lettuce and radicchio in a serving bowl. Place the shrimp mixture on top, toss, and serve.

VARY IT! Pan-seared scallops and leftover rotisserie chicken would taste great in this salad as well.

PER SERVING: *Choices/Exchanges 1 Nonstarchy Vegetable, 2 Lean Protein, 2 Fat; Calories 200 (from Fat 130); Fat 14g (Saturated 1.9g, Trans 0.0g); Cholesterol 105mg; Sodium 140mg; Potassium 400mg; Total Carbohydrate 5g (Dietary Fiber 1g, Sugars 1g); Protein 15g; Phosphorus 175mg.*

Wild Rice Salad

PREP TIME: ABOUT 5 MIN | COOK TIME: 40–50 MIN | SERVINGS: 6 | SERVING SIZE: ⅔ CUP

INGREDIENTS

1 cup raw wild rice (rinsed)

4 cups cold water

1 cup mandarin oranges, packed in their own juice (drain and reserve 2 tablespoons of liquid)

½ cup chopped celery

¼ cup minced red bell pepper

1 shallot, minced

1 teaspoon minced thyme

2 tablespoons raspberry vinegar

1 tablespoon extra-virgin olive oil

DIRECTIONS

1 Place the rinsed, raw rice and the water in a saucepan. Bring to a boil, lower the heat, cover the pan, and cook for 45–50 minutes until the rice has absorbed the water. Set the rice aside to cool.

2 In a large bowl, combine the mandarin oranges, celery, red pepper, and shallot.

3 In a small bowl, combine the reserved juice, thyme, vinegar, and oil.

4 Add the rice to the mandarin oranges and vegetables. Pour the dressing over the salad, toss, and serve.

VARY IT! Swap out the celery for spinach and the oranges for strawberries when in season for a flavorful change.

PER SERVING: *Choices/Exchanges 1 Starch, ½ Carbohydrate, ½ Fat; Calories 130 (from Fat 20); Fat 2.5g (Saturated 0.4g, Trans 0.0g); Cholesterol 0mg; Sodium 10mg; Potassium 190mg; Total Carbohydrate 24g (Dietary Fiber 3g, Sugars 5g); Protein 4g; Phosphorus 85mg.*

Zucchini, Carrot, and Fennel Salad

PREP TIME: ABOUT 10 MIN	SERVINGS: 8	SERVING SIZE: ½ CUP VEGETABLES PLUS ¼ CUP ROMAINE

INGREDIENTS

2 medium carrots, peeled and julienned

1 medium zucchini, julienned

½ medium fennel bulb, core removed and julienned

1 tablespoon fresh orange juice

2 tablespoons Dijon mustard

3 tablespoons extra-virgin olive oil

1 teaspoon white wine vinegar

½ teaspoon dried thyme

1 tablespoon finely minced parsley

$\frac{1}{16}$ teaspoon salt

¼ teaspoon freshly ground black pepper

¼ cup chopped walnuts

1 medium head romaine lettuce, washed and leaves separated

DIRECTIONS

1 Place the carrots, zucchini, and fennel in a medium bowl; set aside.

2 In a medium bowl, combine the orange juice, mustard, olive oil, vinegar, thyme, parsley, salt, and pepper; mix well.

3 Pour the dressing over the vegetables and toss. Add the walnuts, and mix again. Refrigerate until ready to serve.

4 To serve, line a bowl or plates with lettuce leaves, and spoon ½ cup of salad on top.

VARY IT! Orange-infused olive oil and vinegar would work well in this salad as well.

PER SERVING: *Choices/Exchanges 1 Nonstarchy Vegetable, 1½ Fat; Calories 100 (from Fat 70); Fat 8g (Saturated 1.0g, Trans 0.0g); Cholesterol 0mg; Sodium 130mg; Potassium 320mg; Total Carbohydrate 6g (Dietary Fiber 3g, Sugars 3g); Protein 2g; Phosphorus 55mg.*

Classic Vinaigrette

INGREDIENTS

¾ cup olive oil

3 tablespoons fresh lemon juice

1 garlic clove, minced

2 tablespoons white wine vinegar

2 teaspoons Dijon mustard

1 teaspoon minced fresh parsley

$\frac{1}{16}$ teaspoon salt

$\frac{1}{16}$ teaspoon freshly ground black pepper

DIRECTIONS

1 In a blender or food processor, combine all ingredients.

2 Process until well blended. Refrigerate until ready to use.

VARY IT! Spice up this basic dressing with chopped, fresh herbs such as basil or dill.

PER SERVING: *Choices/Exchanges 2 Fat; Calories 80 (from Fat 80): Fat 9g (Saturated 1.2g, Trans 0.0g); Cholesterol 0mg; Sodium 20mg; Potassium 5mg; Total Carbohydrate 0g (Dietary Fiber 0g; Sugars 0g); Protein 0g; Phosphorus 0mg.*

Creamy Herb Dressing

PREP TIME: ABOUT 5 MIN PLUS CHILLING TIME | SERVINGS: 24 | SERVING SIZE: 1 TABLESPOON

INGREDIENTS

½ cup plain fat-free yogurt

1 cup low-fat cottage cheese

1½ teaspoons fresh lemon juice

1 medium carrot, peeled and grated

2 teaspoons grated onion

½ teaspoon dried thyme

¼ teaspoon dried marjoram

¼ teaspoon dried oregano

¼ teaspoon dried basil

DIRECTIONS

1 In a food processor, combine the yogurt, cottage cheese, and lemon juice; process until smooth. Pour into a small mixing bowl.

2 Add the remaining ingredients, and mix well. Add ¼ teaspoon salt, if desired. Cover, and chill in the refrigerator for 1–2 hours before serving.

TIP: Use this low-fat, low-calorie creamy dressing over salad greens or as a dip for vegetables.

PER SERVING: *Choices/Exchanges Free Food; Calories 10 (from Fat 0); Fat 0g (Saturated 0.1g, Trans 0.0g); Cholesterol 0mg; Sodium 45mg; Potassium 30mg; Total Carbohydrate 1g (Dietary Fiber 0g; Sugars 1g); Protein 1g; Phosphorus 20mg.*

Dill Dressing

PREP TIME: ABOUT 5 MIN PLUS CHILLING TIME | SERVINGS: 16 | SERVING SIZE: 1 TABLESPOON

INGREDIENTS

½ cup plain fat-free yogurt

2 tablespoons low-fat mayonnaise

2 teaspoons grated onion

1 garlic clove, minced

¼ cup fat-free milk

1 teaspoon dried dill or 2 teaspoons chopped fresh dill

¼ teaspoon dried oregano

¼ teaspoon freshly ground black pepper

DIRECTIONS

1 In a food processor or blender, combine all ingredients, and process until smooth.

2 Pour into a container, cover, and chill in the refrigerator for 1–2 hours before serving.

TIP: Try this creamy dressing with fresh grilled salmon, swordfish, another fish, or chicken.

PER SERVING: *Choices/Exchanges Free Food; Calories 10 (from Fat 0); Fat 0g (Saturated 0.0g, Trans 0.0g); Cholesterol 0mg; Sodium 20mg; Potassium 20mg; Total Carbohydrate 1g (Dietary Fiber 0g; Sugars 1g); Protein 1g; Phosphorus 15mg.*

French Dressing

INGREDIENTS

½ cup olive oil

¼ cup malt vinegar

$\frac{1}{16}$ teaspoon lemon pepper

Dash paprika

¼ teaspoon dry mustard

DIRECTIONS

1 In a blender or food processor, combine all ingredients.

2 Add ½ teaspoon salt if desired. Process until well blended. Refrigerate until ready to use.

PER SERVING: *Choices/Exchanges 2 Fat; Calories 80 (from Fat 80); Fat 9g (Saturated 1.2g, Trans 0.0g); Cholesterol 0mg; Sodium 0mg; Potassium 0mg; Total Carbohydrate 0g (Dietary Fiber 0g; Sugars 0g); Protein 0g; Phosphorus 0mg.*

Ginger–Soy Dressing

| PREP TIME: ABOUT 5 MIN | SERVINGS: 10 | SERVING SIZE: 1 TABLESPOON |

INGREDIENTS

¼ cup light or reduced-sodium soy sauce

2 tablespoons sesame oil

2 tablespoons rice vinegar

1 tablespoon grated fresh ginger

1 tablespoon dry sherry

1 teaspoon light agave nectar

DIRECTIONS

1 In a small jar, combine all ingredients. Cover the jar tightly, and shake vigorously until well blended.

2 Keep covered, and refrigerated until ready to serve. Shake again before serving.

TIP: This dressing can double as a marinade for chicken, turkey, or fish.

PER SERVING: *Choices/Exchanges ½ Fat; Calories 35 (from Fat 20); Fat 2.5g (Saturated 0.4g, Trans 0.0g); Cholesterol 0mg; Sodium 220mg; Potassium 15mg; Total Carbohydrate 1g (Dietary Fiber 0g; Sugars 1g); Protein 1g; Phosphorus 10mg.*

Light Hollandaise

PREP TIME: ABOUT 5 MIN | COOK TIME: 3–4 MIN | SERVINGS: 4 | SERVING SIZE: 2 TABLESPOONS

INGREDIENTS

½ cup light mayonnaise

3 tablespoons water

1 tablespoon lemon juice

¼ teaspoon freshly ground white pepper

DIRECTIONS

1 In a small saucepan, combine all ingredients. Whisk until smooth.

2 Simmer the mixture over low heat, stirring constantly, for 3–4 minutes until heated through. Serve over any fresh, lightly steamed vegetable.

PER SERVING: *Choices/Exchanges 1½ Fat; Calories 70 (from Fat 60); Fat 7g (Saturated 0.6g, Trans 0.0g); Cholesterol 7mg; Sodium 230mg; Potassium 15mg; Total Carbohydrate 3g (Dietary Fiber 0g; Sugars 1g); Protein 0g; Phosphorus 5mg.*

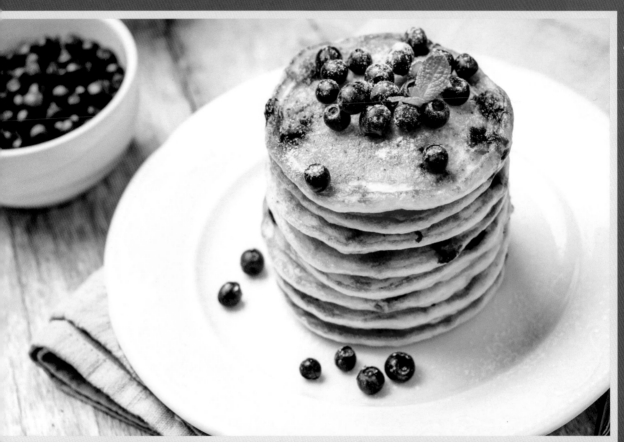

Fresh Blueberry Pancakes (Chapter 4)

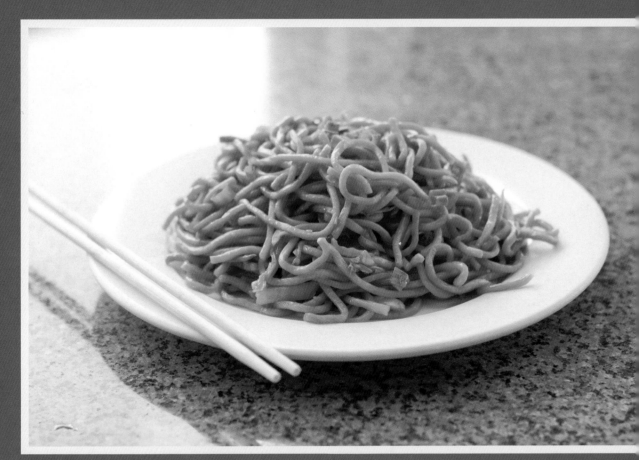

Vegetable Lo Mein (Chapter 6)

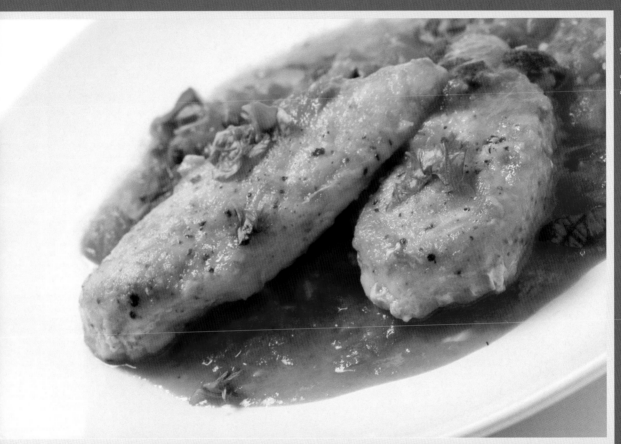

Chicken Provençal (Chapter 7)

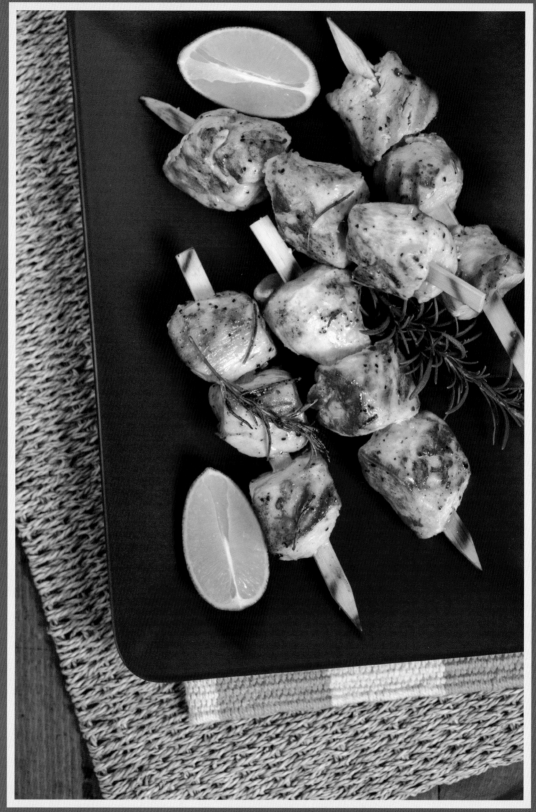

Chicken Kabobs (Chapter 10)

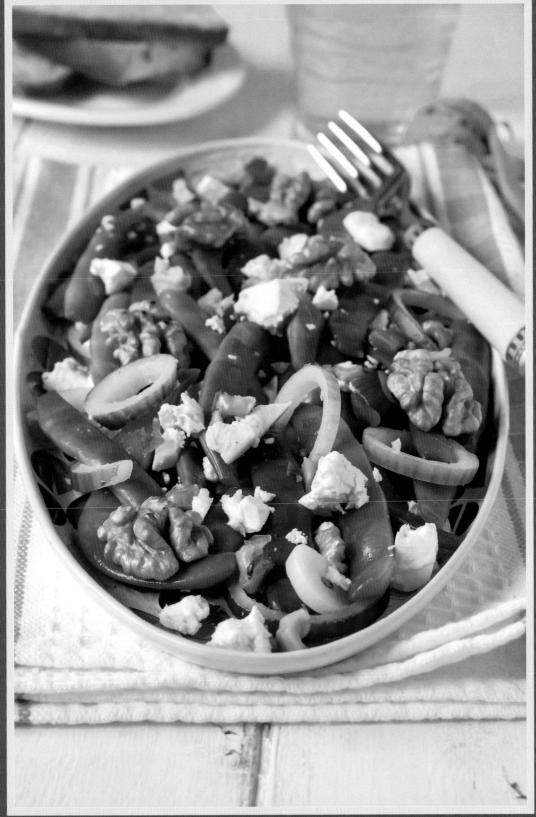

Haricot Verts, Walnut, and Feta Salad (Chapter 11)

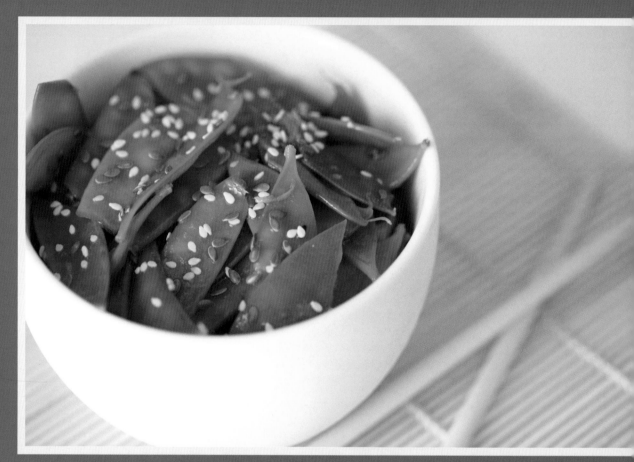

Snow Peas with Sesame Seeds (Chapter 12)

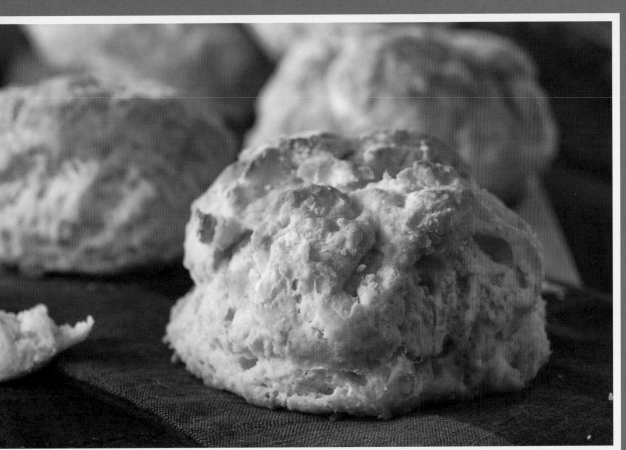

Buttermilk Biscuits (Chapter 14)

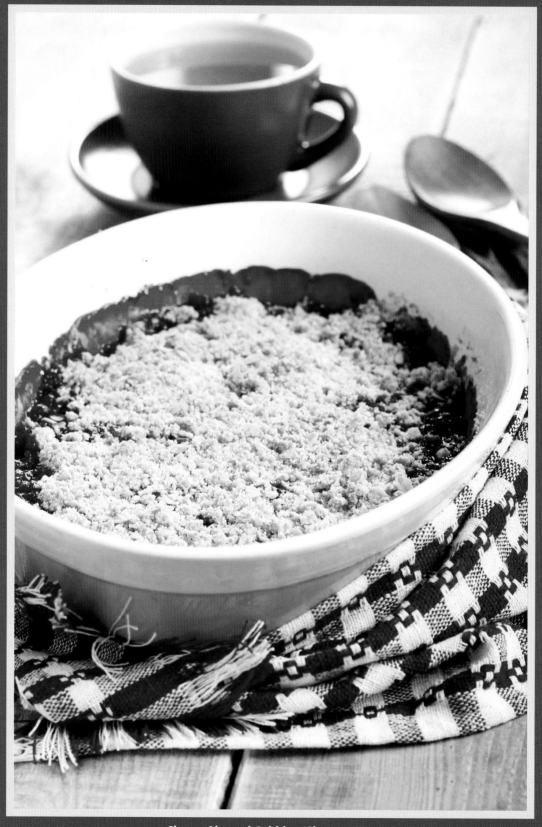

Cherry Almond Cobbler (Chapter 15)

Parmesan Dressing

INGREDIENTS

½ cup white wine vinegar

3 tablespoons Parmesan cheese

1 garlic clove, minced

½ cup olive oil

1 teaspoon dried basil

¼ teaspoon freshly ground black pepper

DIRECTIONS

1 In a jar, combine all ingredients, and cover. Add a dash of salt, if desired.

2 Shake vigorously, and refrigerate until ready to use.

TIP: This dressing also tastes good with cooked broccoli, string beans, or asparagus.

PER SERVING: *Choices/Exchanges 1½ Fat; Calories 60 (from Fat 60); Fat 7g (Saturated 1.0g, Trans 0.0g); Cholesterol 0mg; Sodium 5mg; Potassium 5mg; Total Carbohydrate 0g (Dietary Fiber 0g; Sugars 0g); Protein 0g; Phosphorus 5mg.*

Chapter 12
Vegetables

RECITPES IN THIS CHAPTER

- ⟁ **Artichokes Parmesan**
- ⟁ **Asparagus with Vinaigrette**
- ⟁ **Broccoli with Lemon Sauce**
- ⟁ **Carrots Marsala**
- ⟁ **Chinese Asparagus**
- ⟁ **Green Beans with Garlic and Onion**
- ⟁ **Herb-Broiled Tomatoes**
- **Mushroom Cassoulets**
- ⟁ **Sautéed Sweet Peppers**
- ⟁ **Sherried Peppers with Bean Sprouts**
- ⟁ **Snow Peas with Sesame Seeds**
- ⟁ **Squash and Tomato Cassoulet**
- ⟁ **Vegetable-Stuffed Yellow Squash**
- ⟁ **Zucchini Sauté**

Vegetables are an essential part of a healthy diet. They provide fiber, vitamins, and other beneficial nutrients but are generally low in calories. There are two types of vegetables: nonstarchy vegetables (which are relatively low in carbohydrate) and starchy vegetables (which are higher in carbohydrate). Nonstarchy vegetables — such as tomatoes, onions, mushrooms, carrots, broccoli, peppers, and green beans — are the best vegetable choices for people with diabetes. They nourish the body, and you should include several servings of these vegetables in your meal plan. Starchy vegetables — such as white potatoes, sweet potatoes, corn, and green peas — still have nutritional benefits but should be enjoyed in moderation. For more information on starchy and nonstarchy vegetables, see Chapter 1.

If you're not used to eating a lot of vegetables, don't be intimidated. Incorporating vegetables into your meal plan doesn't mean you have to eat a lot of salads and bland steamed veggies. The recipes in this chapter combine delicious ingredients with healthy cooking methods to enhance the natural flavors of nonstarchy vegetables, creating incredibly satisfying dishes. You might think of vegetables as side dishes, but you can also enjoy vegetable dishes as entrées. Try replacing the animal-based protein in your meal with one of the heartier recipes in this chapter, such as Artichokes Parmesan or Vegetable-Stuffed Yellow Squash. If you're feeling adventurous, you can make a meatless meal one or two nights a week!

Artichokes Parmesan

PREP TIME: ABOUT 5 MIN	COOK TIME: 20 MIN	SERVINGS: 6	SERVING SIZE: ⅓ CUP

INGREDIENTS

½ cup dried whole-wheat bread crumbs

2 tablespoons grated Parmigiano-Reggiano cheese

⅛ teaspoon freshly ground black pepper

9 ounces frozen artichoke hearts, thawed

2 tablespoons extra-virgin olive oil, divided

2 medium tomatoes, diced

DIRECTIONS

1 Preheat the oven to 425 degrees.

2 In a small bowl, combine the bread crumbs, cheese, and black pepper, and stir to combine.

3 Arrange the artichoke hearts in a 1-quart casserole dish. Sprinkle the tomatoes over the top. Season with salt, if desired.

4 Sprinkle the bread crumb mixture over the vegetables, and bake for 15–20 minutes or until the topping is light brown.

VARY IT! Zucchini slices could also be prepared this way.

PER SERVING: *Choices/Exchanges ½ Starch, 1 Nonstarchy Vegetable, 1 Fat; Calories 100 (from Fat 45); Fat 5g (Saturated 1.1g, Trans 0.0g); Cholesterol 0mg; Sodium 50mg; Potassium 240mg; Total Carbohydrate 11g (Dietary Fiber 4g; Sugars 2g); Protein 3g; Phosphorus 60mg.*

Asparagus with Vinaigrette

PREP TIME: ABOUT 5 MIN | COOK TIME: 10 MIN | SERVINGS: 6 | SERVING SIZE: ½ CUP

INGREDIENTS

1½ pounds fresh or frozen asparagus (thin pieces)

½ cup red wine vinegar

½ teaspoon dried or 1 teaspoon fresh tarragon

2 tablespoons finely chopped fresh chives

3 tablespoons finely chopped fresh parsley

½ cup water

1 tablespoon extra-virgin olive oil

1⅓ tablespoons Dijon mustard

1 pound fresh spinach leaves, trimmed of stems, washed, and dried

2 large tomatoes, cut into wedges

DIRECTIONS

1 Place 1 inch of water in a pot, and place a steamer inside. Arrange the asparagus on top of the steamer. Steam fresh asparagus for 4 minutes or frozen asparagus for 6–8 minutes. Immediately rinse the asparagus under cold water to stop the cooking. (This helps keep asparagus bright green and crunchy.) Set aside.

2 In a small bowl or salad cruet, combine the remaining ingredients except the spinach and tomatoes. Mix, or shake well.

3 To serve, line plates with the spinach leaves, and place the asparagus on top of the spinach. Garnish with the tomato wedges, and spoon any remaining dressing on top.

PER SERVING: *Choices/Exchanges 2 Nonstarchy Vegetable, ½ Fat; Calories 80 (from Fat 25); Fat 3g (Saturated 0.4g, Trans 0.0g); Cholesterol 0mg; Sodium 150mg; Potassium 770mg; Total Carbohydrate 10g (Dietary Fiber 4g; Sugars 3g); Protein 5g; Phosphorus 105mg.*

Broccoli with Lemon Sauce

PREP TIME: ABOUT 5 MIN	COOK TIME: 10 MIN	SERVINGS: 16	SERVING SIZE: ½ CUP

INGREDIENTS

1½ pounds fresh broccoli florets

2 tablespoons extra-virgin olive oil

2 tablespoons fresh lemon juice

Zest of 1 lemon

¼ teaspoon kosher salt

⅛ teaspoon freshly ground black pepper

1 large lemon, cut into wedges

DIRECTIONS

1 Place the broccoli in a vegetable steamer basket over boiling water. Cover, and simmer for 8–10 minutes until broccoli is just tender.

2 Transfer the broccoli to a serving bowl. Drizzle the olive oil and lemon juice over the broccoli. Garnish with the lemon zest, salt, and pepper, and serve with lemon wedges.

PER SERVING: *Choices/Exchanges 1 Nonstarchy Vegetable; Calories 30 (from Fat 20); Fat 2g (Saturated 0.3g, Trans 0.0g); Cholesterol 0mg; Sodium 45mg; Potassium 140mg; Total Carbohydrate 3g (Dietary Fiber 1g; Sugars 1g); Protein 1g, Phosphorus 30mg.*

Carrots Marsala

PREP TIME: ABOUT 5 MIN | COOK TIME: 10 MIN | SERVINGS: 6 | SERVING SIZE: ½ CUP

INGREDIENTS

10 carrots (about 1 pound), peeled and diagonally sliced

¼ cup Marsala wine

¼ cup water

1 tablespoon extra-virgin olive oil

⅛ teaspoon freshly ground black pepper

1 tablespoon finely chopped fresh parsley

DIRECTIONS

1 In a large saucepan, combine the carrots, wine, water, oil, and pepper. Bring to a boil, cover, reduce the heat, and simmer for 8–10 minutes, until the carrots are just tender, basting occasionally. Taste, and add salt, if desired.

2 Transfer to a serving dish, spoon any juices on top, and sprinkle with parsley.

PER SERVING: *Choices/Exchanges 1 Nonstarchy Vegetable, ½ Fat; Calories 60 (from Fat 20); Fat 2.5g (Saturated 0.3g, Trans 0.0g); Cholesterol 0mg; Sodium 45mg; Potassium 220mg; Total Carbohydrate 7g (Dietary Fiber 2g; Sugars 4g); Protein 1g; Phosphorus 25mg.*

Chinese Asparagus

INGREDIENTS

1 pound asparagus

½ cup plus 1 tablespoon water, divided

1 tablespoon light soy sauce

1 tablespoon rice vinegar

2 teaspoons cornstarch

1 tablespoon canola oil

2 teaspoons grated fresh ginger

1 scallion, minced

DIRECTIONS

1 Trim the tough ends off the asparagus. Cut the stalks diagonally into 2-inch pieces.

2 In a small bowl, combine the ½ cup water, soy sauce, and rice vinegar.

3 In a measuring cup, combine the cornstarch and 1 tablespoon water. Set aside.

4 Heat the oil in a wok or skillet. Add the ginger and scallions, and stir-fry for 30 seconds. Add the asparagus and stir-fry for a few seconds more. Add the broth mixture, and bring to a boil. Cover, and simmer for 3–5 minutes, until the asparagus is just tender.

5 Add the cornstarch mixture, and cook until thickened. Serve.

PER SERVING: *Choices/Exchanges 1 Nonstarchy Vegetable, ½ Fat; Calories 50 (from Fat 30); Fat 3.5g (Saturated 0.3g, Trans 0.0g); Cholesterol 0mg; Sodium 140mg; Potassium 140mg; Total Carbohydrate 5g (Dietary Fiber 1g; Sugars 1g); Protein 2g; Phosphorus 40mg.*

Green Beans with Garlic and Onion

PREP TIME: ABOUT 5 MIN | COOK TIME: 12 MIN | SERVINGS: 8 | SERVING SIZE: ½ CUP

INGREDIENTS

1 pound fresh green beans, trimmed and cut into 2-inch pieces

1 tablespoon extra-virgin olive oil

1 small onion, chopped

1 large garlic clove, minced

1 tablespoon white vinegar

¼ cup Parmigiano-Reggiano cheese

⅛ teaspoon freshly ground black pepper

DIRECTIONS

1 Steam the beans for 7 minutes or until just tender. Set aside.

2 In a skillet, heat the oil over low heat. Add the onion and garlic, and sauté for 4–5 minutes or until the onion is translucent.

3 Transfer the beans to a serving bowl, and add the onion mixture and vinegar, tossing well. Sprinkle with cheese and pepper, and serve.

PER SERVING: *Choices/Exchanges 1 Nonstarchy Vegetable, ½ Fat; Calories 50 (from Fat 20); Fat 2.5g (Saturated 0.8g, Trans 0.0g); Cholesterol 3mg; Sodium 15mg; Potassium 95mg; Total Carbohydrate 5g (Dietary Fiber 2g; Sugars 1g); Protein 2g; Phosphorus 35mg.*

Herb–Broiled Tomatoes

PREP TIME: ABOUT 5 MIN	COOK TIME: 5–10 MIN	SERVINGS: 8	SERVING SIZE: ½ TOMATO

INGREDIENTS

4 medium tomatoes

¼ cup Parmigiano-Reggiano cheese

2 tablespoons dried bread crumbs

2 tablespoons minced fresh parsley

1 teaspoon minced fresh basil

1 teaspoon minced fresh oregano

⅛ teaspoon freshly ground black pepper

1 tablespoon extra-virgin olive oil

DIRECTIONS

1 Remove the stems from the tomatoes, and cut in half crosswise.

2 In a small bowl, combine the remaining ingredients, and lightly press the mixture over the cut sides of the tomato halves.

3 Place the tomatoes on a baking sheet, cut side up, and broil about 6 inches from the heat for 3–5 minutes or until the topping is browned.

PER SERVING: *Choices/Exchanges 1 Nonstarchy Vegetable, ½ Fat; Calories 45 (from Fat 20); Fat 2.5g (Saturated 0.8g, Trans 0.0g); Cholesterol 3mg; Sodium 35mg; Potassium 190mg; Total Carbohydrate 4g (Dietary Fiber 1g; Sugars 2g); Protein 2g; Phosphorus 40mg.*

Mushroom Cassoulets

| PREP TIME: ABOUT 5 MIN | COOK TIME: 30 MIN | SERVINGS: 6 | SERVING SIZE: ½ CUP |

INGREDIENTS

1 pound mushrooms, sliced

½ cup lentils, cooked

1 medium onion, chopped

1 cup low-sodium chicken broth

1 sprig thyme

1 bay leaf

Leaves from 1 celery stalk

2 tablespoons lemon juice

⅛ teaspoon freshly ground black pepper

½ cup wheat germ

2 tablespoons extra-virgin olive oil

DIRECTIONS

1 Preheat the oven to 350 degrees.

2 In a saucepan, combine the mushrooms, lentils, onion, and chicken broth. Tie together the thyme, bay leaf, and celery leaves and add to the mushrooms.

3 Add the lemon juice and pepper, and bring to a boil. Boil until the liquid is reduced, about 10 minutes. Remove the bundle of herbs.

4 Divide the mushroom mixture equally into small ramekins. Mix the wheat germ and oil together, and sprinkle on top of each casserole.

5 Bake at 350 degrees for 20 minutes or until the tops are golden brown. Remove from the oven, and let cool slightly before serving. Add salt if desired.

PER SERVING: *Choices/Exchanges ½ Starch, 1 Nonstarchy Vegetable, 1 Fat; Calories 130 (from Fat 50); Fat 6g (Saturated 0.9g, Trans 0.0g); Cholesterol 0mg; Sodium 30mg; Potassium 470mg; Total Carbohydrate 13g (Dietary Fiber 4g; Sugars 4g); Protein 8g; Phosphorus 220mg.*

Sautéed Sweet Peppers

PREP TIME: ABOUT 5 MIN	COOK TIME: 10 MIN	SERVINGS: 6	SERVING SIZE: ½ CUP VEGETABLES AND ⅓ CUP RICE

INGREDIENTS

1 tablespoon extra-virgin olive oil

2 medium green bell peppers, cut into 1-inch squares

2 medium red bell peppers, cut into 1-inch squares

2 tablespoons water

¼ teaspoon salt

⅛ teaspoon freshly ground black pepper

2 tablespoons finely chopped fresh basil or oregano

2 cups precooked brown rice, hot

DIRECTIONS

1 In a large skillet over medium heat, heat the oil. Add the peppers, and sauté for 3–5 minutes, stirring frequently.

2 Add the water, salt, and pepper; continue sautéing for 4–5 minutes or until the peppers are just tender. Stir in the basil, and remove from the heat.

3 Spread the rice over a serving platter, spoon the peppers and liquid on top, and serve.

VARY IT! Zucchini, squash, and mushrooms can all be prepared in addition to or instead of the peppers in this dish.

PER SERVING: *Choices/Exchanges 1 Starch, 1 Nonstarchy Vegetable, ½ Fat; Calories 130 (from Fat 25); Fat 3g (Saturated 0.5g, Trans 0.0g); Cholesterol 0mg; Sodium 105mg; Potassium 250mg; Total Carbohydrate 22g (Dietary Fiber 3g; Sugars 3g); Protein 3g; Phosphorus 90mg.*

Sherried Peppers with Bean Sprouts

PREP TIME: ABOUT 5 MIN	COOK TIME: 7–10 MIN	SERVINGS: 4	SERVING SIZE: ½ CUP

INGREDIENTS

1 green bell pepper, julienned

1 red bell pepper, julienned

2 cups canned, drained bean sprouts

2 teaspoons light soy sauce

1 tablespoon dry sherry

1 teaspoon red wine vinegar

DIRECTIONS

1 In a large skillet over medium heat, combine the peppers, bean sprouts, soy sauce, and sherry, mixing well. Cover, and cook 5–7 minutes, until the vegetables are just tender.

2 Stir in the vinegar, and remove from the heat. Serve hot.

VARY IT! This side dish has so many options. You can add carrots, snow peas, or broccoli for more vegetables, or serve over rice, noodles, or even a baked sweet potato.

PER SERVING: *Choices/Exchanges 1 Nonstarchy Vegetable; Calories 30 (from Fat 0); Fat 0g (Saturated 0.0g, Trans 0.0g); Cholesterol 0mg; Sodium 120mg; Potassium 170mg; Total Carbohydrate 6g (Dietary Fiber 2g; Sugars 3g); Protein 2g; Phosphorus 40mg.*

Snow Peas with Sesame Seeds

PREP TIME: ABOUT 5 MIN	COOK TIME: 5 MIN	SERVINGS: 6	SERVING SIZE: ½ CUP

INGREDIENTS

2 cups water

1 pound trimmed fresh snow peas

3 tablespoons sesame seeds

1 tablespoon chopped shallots

¼ teaspoon salt

⅛ teaspoon freshly ground black pepper

1 teaspoon ground ginger

DIRECTIONS

1 In a saucepan over high heat, boil the water. Add the snow peas, and then turn off the heat. After 1 minute, rinse the snow peas under cold running water to stop the cooking process; drain. (This method of blanching helps the snow peas to retain their bright green color and crispness.)

2 In a skillet, toast the sesame seeds for 1 minute over medium heat. Add the snow peas, shallots, salt, pepper, and ginger. Continue sautéing for 1–2 minutes until the snow peas are coated with sesame seeds. Serve.

TIP: Try these crisp snow peas with Sea Bass with Ginger Sauce (see Chapter 9).

PER SERVING: *Choices/Exchanges 1 Nonstarchy Vegetable, ½ Fat; Calories 50 (from Fat 20); Fat 2g (Saturated 0.3g, Trans 0.0g); Cholesterol 0mg; Sodium 100mg; Potassium 170mg; Total Carbohydrate 7g (Dietary Fiber 2g; Sugars 3g); Protein 3g; Phosphorus 65mg.*

Squash and Tomato Cassoulet

PREP TIME: ABOUT 5 MIN | COOK TIME: 30 MIN | SERVINGS: 6 | SERVING SIZE: ½ CUP

INGREDIENTS

1 tablespoon extra-virgin olive oil

6 small yellow squash, sliced

1 medium onion, minced

2 garlic cloves, minced

2 tablespoons chopped fresh parsley

¼ teaspoon salt

⅛ teaspoon freshly ground black pepper

2 medium tomatoes, sliced

3 egg whites

1 cup fat-free milk

DIRECTIONS

1 Preheat the oven to 350 degrees.

2 In a large skillet over medium heat, heat the oil. Add the squash, onion, and garlic, and sauté for 5 minutes. Add the parsley, salt, and pepper.

3 Layer the squash mixture and tomatoes in a casserole dish.

4 In a bowl, combine the egg whites and milk, blending well. Pour over the vegetables.

5 Bake at 350 degrees for 20–25 minutes or until the custard is set. Remove from the oven, and let cool slightly before serving.

PER SERVING: Choices/Exchanges 2 Nonstarchy Vegetable, ½ Fat; Calories 80 (from Fat 20); Fat 2.5g (Saturated 0.4g, Trans 0.0g); Cholesterol 0mg; Sodium 150mg; Potassium 560mg; Total Carbohydrate 11g (Dietary Fiber 2g; Sugars 7g); Protein 5g; Phosphorus 110mg.

Vegetable-Stuffed Yellow Squash

PREP TIME: ABOUT 10 MIN	COOK TIME: 30 MIN	SERVINGS: 6	SERVING SIZE: 1 SQUASH

INGREDIENTS

6 small yellow squash

1 tomato, finely chopped

½ cup minced onion

½ cup finely chopped green bell pepper

½ cup shredded 50 percent reduced-fat sharp cheddar

¼ teaspoon salt

⅛ teaspoon freshly ground black pepper

DIRECTIONS

1 Preheat the oven to 400 degrees.

2 Place the squash in a large pot of boiling water. Cover, reduce heat, and simmer for 5–7 minutes or until the squash is just tender. Drain, and allow to cool slightly.

3 Trim the stems from the squash, and cut in half lengthwise. Gently scoop out the pulp, leaving a firm shell. Drain, and chop the pulp.

4 In a large mixing bowl, combine the pulp and the remaining ingredients, blending well.

5 Place the squash shells in a 13-x-9-x-2-inch baking dish, gently spoon the vegetable mixture into the shells, and bake at 400 degrees for 15–20 minutes. Remove from the oven, and let cool slightly before serving.

PER SERVING: *CHOICES/EXCHANGES 1 Nonstarchy Vegetable, ½ Fat; Calories 60 (from Fat 20); Fat 2g (Saturated 1.1g, Trans 0.0g); Cholesterol 2mg; Sodium 160mg; Potassium 430mg; Total Carbohydrate 7g (Dietary Fiber 2g; Sugars 4g); Protein 5g; Phosphorus 105mg.*

Zucchini Sauté

| PREP TIME: ABOUT 5 MIN | COOK TIME: 10 MIN | SERVINGS: 4 | SERVING SIZE: ½ CUP |

INGREDIENTS

1 tablespoon olive oil

1 medium red onion, finely chopped

3 medium zucchini (about 5–6 ounces each), cut into ¼-inch thick rounds

¼ teaspoon dried oregano

⅛ teaspoon salt

⅛ teaspoon freshly ground black pepper

DIRECTIONS

1 In a large skillet over medium heat, heat the oil. Add the onion, and sauté until the onion is translucent but not browned.

2 Add the zucchini, cover, and simmer 3–4 minutes. Sprinkle with the oregano, salt, and pepper, and serve hot.

PER SERVING: *Choices/Exchanges 1 Nonstarchy Vegetable, 1 Fat; Calories 60 (from Fat 35); Fat 4g (Saturated 0.6g, Trans 0.0g); Cholesterol 0mg; Sodium 85mg; Potassium 340mg; Total Carbohydrate 7g (Dietary Fiber 2g; Sugars 4g); Protein 2g; Phosphorus 50mg.*

Chapter **13**
Rice and Potatoes

RECIPES IN THIS CHAPTER

Rice and potato side dishes can be a great addition to healthy meals! They're warm and hearty, and add a touch of comfort to even the simplest of meals. Some people think you need to avoid all starchy foods if you have diabetes. Although it's true that starchy foods — bread, pasta, grains, beans, potatoes, and corn, for example — are relatively high in carbohydrate, they can still be part of a diabetes meal plan. The trick is to choose the most nutrient-rich options when adding starchy foods to your plate. Look for whole grains, beans, and starchy vegetables instead of processed starches.

The recipes in this chapter showcase the versatility and richness of nutritious starches such as brown rice and white and sweet potatoes. Rice and potatoes are a perfect canvas for many different flavor profiles — from classic American and Mediterranean to a variety of exotic Asian flavors. These easy-to-prepare dishes will soon be favorites in your home!

Asian Fried Rice

PREP TIME: ABOUT 5 MIN | COOK TIME: 20 MIN | SERVINGS: 4 | SERVING SIZE: ½ CUP

INGREDIENTS

2 tablespoons peanut oil

¼ cup chopped onion

1 cup sliced carrot

1 green bell pepper, diced

1 tablespoon grated fresh ginger

2 cups cooked brown rice, cold

½ cup water chestnuts, drained

½ cup sliced mushrooms

1 tablespoon light soy sauce

2 egg whites

½ cup sliced scallions

DIRECTIONS

1 In a large skillet, heat the oil. Sauté the onion, carrot, green pepper, and ginger for 5–6 minutes.

2 Stir in the rice, water chestnuts, mushrooms, and soy sauce, and stir-fry for 8–10 minutes.

3 Stir in the egg whites, and continue to stir-fry for another 3 minutes. Top with the sliced scallions to serve.

TIP: Prep the vegetables in advance to speed up the cooking time.

VARY IT! Leftover pieces of chicken, turkey breast, and grilled vegetables added to this side dish can transform it into an entrée.

PER SERVING: Choices/Exchanges 1½ Starch, 2 Nonstarchy Vegetable, 1 Fat; Calories 220 (from Fat 70); Fat 8g (Saturated 1.4g, Trans 0.0g); Cholesterol 0mg; Sodium 200mg; Potassium 380mg; Total Carbohydrate 32g (Dietary Fiber 4g; Sugars 4g); Protein 6g; Phosphorus 135mg.

Colorful Rice Casserole

PREP TIME: ABOUT 5 MIN	COOK TIME: 20 MIN	SERVINGS: 12	SERVING SIZE: ¼ CUP RICE AND ½ CUP VEGETABLES

INGREDIENTS

1 tablespoon extra-virgin olive oil

1½ pounds zucchini, thinly sliced

¾ cup chopped scallions

2 cups corn kernels (frozen or fresh; if frozen, defrost)

One 14.5-ounce can no-salt-added chopped tomatoes, undrained

¼ cup chopped parsley

1 teaspoon oregano

3 cups cooked brown (or white) rice

⅛ teaspoon freshly ground black pepper

DIRECTIONS

1 In a large skillet, heat the oil. Add the zucchini and scallions, and sauté for 5 minutes.

2 Add the remaining ingredients, cover, reduce heat, and simmer for 10–15 minutes or until the vegetables are heated through. Season with salt, if desired, and pepper. Transfer to a bowl, and serve.

VARY IT! Other types of nonstarchy vegetables such as peppers and eggplants would also work well in this dish.

PER SERVING: *Choices/Exchanges 1 Starch, 1 Nonstarchy Vegetable; Calories 110 (from Fat 20); Fat 2g (Saturated 0.4g, Trans 0.0g); Cholesterol 0mg; Sodium 20mg; Potassium 330mg; Total Carbohydrate 21g (Dietary Fiber 2g; Sugars 4g); Protein 3g; Phosphorus 100mg.*

Curried Rice with Pineapple

PREP TIME: ABOUT 5 MIN PLUS SOAKING TIME	COOK TIME: 35 MIN	SERVINGS: 8	SERVING SIZE: ⅓ CUP

INGREDIENTS

1 onion, chopped

1½ cups water

1¼ cups low-sodium chicken broth

1 cup uncooked brown basmati rice, soaked in water 20 minutes and drained before cooking

2 red bell peppers, minced

1 teaspoon curry powder

1 teaspoon ground turmeric

1 teaspoon ground ginger

2 garlic cloves, minced

One 8-ounce can pineapple chunks packed in juice, drained

¼ cup sliced almonds, toasted

DIRECTIONS

1 In a medium saucepan, combine the onion, water, and chicken broth. Bring to a boil, and add the rice, peppers, curry powder, turmeric, ginger, and garlic. Cover, placing a paper towel in between the pot and the lid, and reduce the heat. Simmer for 25 minutes.

2 Add the pineapple, and continue to simmer 5–7 minutes more until rice is tender and water is absorbed. Taste and add salt, if desired. Transfer to a serving bowl, and garnish with almonds to serve.

TIP: Placing a paper towel in between the lid, and the pot helps to absorb the excess steam created by cooking the dish and makes the rice much fluffier.

VARY IT! Quinoa can be replaced for the brown basmati rice to up the protein quotient in this recipe.

PER SERVING: *Choices/Exchanges 1 Starch, 1 Nonstarchy Vegetable, ½ Fat; Calories 130 (from Fat 20); Fat 2.5g (Saturated 0.3g, Trans 0.0g); Cholesterol 0mg; Sodium 25mg; Potassium 250mg; Total Carbohydrate 25g (Dietary Fiber 3g, Sugars 6g); Protein 4g; Phosphorus 120mg.*

Festive Sweet Potatoes

PREP TIME: ABOUT 5 MIN | COOK TIME: 30 MIN | SERVINGS: 8 | SERVING SIZE: ½ CUP

INGREDIENTS

4 sweet potatoes (about 20 ounces total), washed and cubed

2 cups crushed pineapple in its own juice

2 teaspoons cinnamon

1 teaspoon freshly grated nutmeg

1 teaspoon extra-virgin olive oil

2 tablespoons ground flax seeds

1 tablespoon slivered almonds

DIRECTIONS

1 In a large saucepan, boil the potatoes over medium heat for about 10 minutes until you can pierce them easily with a fork (or bake them directly on a rack in a preheated 350-degree oven for 45 minutes).

2 Preheat the oven to 350 degrees. Let the potatoes cool; then gently peel them. Mash the potatoes with the pineapple and spices and place in a casserole dish coated with olive oil.

3 Top the casserole with flax seeds and almonds and bake for 20 minutes, or until the top is golden.

VARY IT! Rutabaga, turnips, carrots, and yucca can be used in place or in addition to the sweet potatoes in this recipe.

PER SERVING: *Choices/Exchanges 1 Starch, ½ Fruit; Calories 110 (from Fat 20); Fat 2.5g (Saturated 0.3g, Trans 0.0g); Cholesterol 0mg; Sodium 20mg; Potassium 340mg; Total Carbohydrate 20g (Dietary Fiber 4g, Sugars 9g); Protein 2g; Phosphorus 55mg.*

Sweet Potato Parmesan Chips

PREP TIME: ABOUT 5 MIN	COOK TIME: 20 MIN	SERVINGS: 4	SERVING SIZE: ABOUT 8 POTATO SLICES

INGREDIENTS

4 large sweet potatoes (5 ounces each)

Nonstick cooking spray

2 tablespoons extra-virgin olive oil

1 teaspoon grated onion

¼ teaspoon sea salt

⅛ teaspoon freshly ground black pepper

¼ teaspoons paprika

2 tablespoons grated Parmigiano-Reggiano cheese

DIRECTIONS

1 Preheat the oven to 425 degrees.

2 Wash and cut the unpeeled potatoes into ⅛-inch-thick slices. Place in a single layer over baking sheets coated with cooking spray.

3 In a small skillet, heat the olive oil, and add the onion, salt, pepper, and paprika. Brush the potatoes with the oil mixture and bake for 15–20 minutes or until the potatoes are crispy and golden brown.

4 Remove from the oven, and sprinkle with cheese. Serve hot.

VARY IT! Try using yellow potatoes and thinly sliced beets in this recipe as well.

PER SERVING: *Choices/Exchanges 1½ Starch, 1½ Fat; Calories 170 (from Fat 70); Fat 8g (Saturated 1.5g, Trans 0.0g); Cholesterol 8mg; Sodium 190mg; Potassium 550mg; Total Carbohydrate 24g (Dietary Fiber 4g, Sugars 8g); Protein 3g; Phosphorus 80mg.*

Rice with Spinach and Feta

INGREDIENTS

¾ cup uncooked brown rice

1½ cups water

1 tablespoon extra-virgin olive oil

1 medium onion, diced

1 cup sliced mushrooms

2 garlic cloves, minced

1 tablespoon lemon juice

½ teaspoon dried oregano

9 cups fresh spinach, stems trimmed, washed, patted dry, and coarsely chopped

⅓ cup crumbled fat-free feta cheese

⅛ teaspoon freshly ground black pepper

DIRECTIONS

1 In a medium saucepan over medium heat, combine the rice and water. Bring to a boil, cover, reduce heat, and simmer for 15 minutes. Transfer to a serving bowl.

2 In a skillet, heat the oil. Sauté the onion, mushrooms, and garlic for 5–7 minutes. Stir in the lemon juice and oregano. Add the spinach, cheese, and pepper, tossing until the spinach is slightly wilted.

3 Toss with rice and serve.

VARY IT! Millet and barley make great substitutions for the rice in this dish. Baby kale can also be used in place of the spinach.

PER SERVING: *Choices/Exchanges 1½ Starch, 1 Nonstarchy Vegetable, ½ Fat; Calories 170 (from Fat 35); Fat 4g (Saturated 0.6g, Trans 0.0g); Cholesterol 0mg; Sodium 115mg; Potassium 470mg; Total Carbohydrate 28g (Dietary Fiber 3g, Sugars 2g); Protein 6g; Phosphorus 160mg.*

Herbed Skillet Potatoes

PREP TIME: ABOUT 5 MIN | COOK TIME: 20 MIN | SERVINGS: 4 | SERVING SIZE: ½ CUP

INGREDIENTS

2 tablespoons extra-virgin olive oil

1 small onion, chopped

1 garlic clove, minced

6 sage leaves, finely chopped

½ teaspoon finely chopped fresh rosemary

2 potatoes (5 ounces each), unpeeled, halved lengthwise, and sliced crosswise into thin slices

3 tablespoons crushed wheat germ

¼ teaspoon sea salt

⅛ teaspoon freshly ground black pepper

DIRECTIONS

1 In a large skillet over medium heat, heat the oil. Add the onion, and garlic and sauté for 2–3 minutes.

2 Add the sage, rosemary, and potatoes. Cover, and cook for 10 minutes, stirring occasionally.

3 Turn the potatoes over with a spatula, season with the wheat germ, salt, and pepper, and continue to cook for another 5–7 minutes until golden brown. Serve.

VARY IT! Cauliflower and broccoli taste great when prepared this way as well.

PER SERVING: *Choices/Exchanges 1 Starch, 1½ Fat; Calories 140 (from Fat 60); Fat 7g (Saturated 1.1g, Trans 0.0g); Cholesterol 0mg; Sodium 140mg; Potassium 400mg; Total Carbohydrate 17g (Dietary Fiber 3g, Sugars 2g); Protein 3g; Phosphorus 110mg.*

Mediterranean-Style Scalloped Potatoes

| PREP TIME: ABOUT 5 MIN | COOK TIME: 45 MIN | SERVINGS: 8 | SERVING SIZE: ½ CUP |

INGREDIENTS

6 small potatoes (4 ounces each), unpeeled, washed, and sliced into ¼-inch-thick slices

4 cups water

1 teaspoon extra-virgin olive oil

⅓ cup chopped onion

1 cup plain low-fat Greek yogurt

Juice and zest of 1 lemon

¼ cup finely chopped baby dill

2 tablespoons crushed flax seeds

¼ teaspoon salt

⅛ teaspoon freshly ground black pepper

DIRECTIONS

1 Preheat the oven to 425 degrees.

2 Place the potatoes in a saucepan with water to cover. Bring to a boil, lower the heat, and let the potatoes cook for 15 minutes, or until fork-tender. Drain the potatoes, and let cool.

3 In a skillet, heat the olive oil. Add the onion, and sauté for 5 minutes.

4 In a bowl, place the Greek yogurt, lemon juice and zest, dill, flax seeds, salt, and pepper; add the onion, and mix well.

5 Lay the potato slices in a casserole dish. Spoon the yogurt mixture over the potatoes.

6 Roast the potatoes for 15–20 minutes, or until the top is browned.

VARY IT! Sweet potatoes can also be used in this dish.

PER SERVING: *Choices/Exchanges 1½ Starch; Calories 120 (from Fat 20); Fat 2.5g (Saturated 0.5g, Trans 0.0g); Cholesterol 0mg; Sodium 90mg; Potassium 400mg; Total Carbohydrate 20g (Dietary Fiber 3g, Sugars 2g); Protein 5g; Phosphorus 95mg.*

Chapter **14**

Breads and Muffins

RECIPES IN THIS CHAPTER

Warm, fragrant breads and muffins make wonderful breakfasts, desserts, and snacks. Many people with diabetes think they need to avoid these delicious treats because of their high carbohydrate content, but the key is to watch your portion sizes and account for these foods in your meal plan. Baked goods can actually be an opportunity to add more fiber, fruits, and even nonstarchy vegetables to your diet. The diabetes-friendly bread and muffin recipes in this chapter incorporate healthy ingredients so you can indulge without derailing your blood glucose–control efforts.

In this chapter, whole-wheat or whole-grain flour is used to replace some or all of the all-purpose flour used in traditional baked goods, which can increase the fiber content. Fruits and vegetables impart rich flavors, amazing texture, and added nutrients to many of the recipes. Whether you're in the mood for a classic muffin or biscuit or a more creative recipe, this chapter has a tasty, comforting bread or muffin recipe for you!

TIP

With a few simple tricks you can make a healthier version of your favorite bread or muffin recipe:

>> Take a lesson from the recipes in this chapter, and try using a whole-grain flour to replace some or all of the white flour in the recipe.

>> Make the most of your baked goods by adding fruits, vegetables, or nuts to increase the fiber content and provide other nutrients.

>> Try replacing oil with applesauce or replacing some or all of the sugar in the recipe with a zero-calorie sugar substitute or a baking blend.

Making any of these changes can affect the texture, color, and baking time of breads or muffins, so it may take some experimentation to get things right. But the payoff — hearty, better-for-you breads and muffins — is worth it!

Banana Carrot Muffins

PREP TIME: ABOUT 5 MIN	COOK TIME: 20 MIN	SERVINGS: 12	SERVING SIZE: 1 MUFFIN

INGREDIENTS

1½ cups whole-wheat flour

2 teaspoons baking powder

1 teaspoon baking soda

½ teaspoon nutmeg

Pinch cloves

½ cup bran

2 egg whites

2 tablespoons agave nectar

½ cup low-fat buttermilk

1 cup mashed banana

1 cup grated carrot

1 teaspoon vanilla

DIRECTIONS

1 Preheat the oven to 400 degrees. In a large bowl, combine the flour, baking powder, baking soda, nutmeg, cloves, and bran.

2 In a smaller bowl, combine the remaining ingredients.

3 Combine all ingredients together, and mix well, but do not overbeat.

4 Spoon into muffin cups lined with paper liners, and bake for 20 minutes at 400 degrees. Serve warm or at room temperature.

PER SERVING: *Choices/Exchanges: 1½ Carbohydrate; Calories 100 (from Fat 5); Fat 0.5g (Saturated 0.2g, Trans 0.0g); Cholesterol 0mg; Sodium 190mg; Potassium 210mg, Total Carbohydrate 21g (Dietary Fiber 4g, Sugars 6g); Protein 4g; Phosphorus 170mg.*

Blueberry Scones

INGREDIENTS

½ cup low-fat buttermilk at room temperature

¾ cup orange juice

Zest of 1 orange

2¼ cups whole-wheat pastry flour

1 teaspoon baking soda

1 teaspoon cream of tartar

⅓ cup agave nectar

¼ cup canola oil

1 cup fresh or frozen (thawed) blueberries

DIRECTIONS

1 Preheat the oven to 375 degrees. In a small bowl, combine the buttermilk, orange juice, and orange peel. Set aside.

2 In a large bowl, sift together the flour, baking soda, cream of tartar, agave nectar, and canola oil. Mix until well combined.

3 Stir in the buttermilk mixture and blueberries, and mix gently by hand until well combined.

4 Turn the batter onto a lightly floured cookie sheet, and pat into a circle about ¾ inch thick and 8 inches across. Using a sharp knife, cut the circle into 14 wedges, cutting almost all the way through.

5 Bake for about 20 minutes, or until lightly browned. Cool, and cut completely through the wedges to serve.

VARY IT! Cranberries also work well in this recipe.

PER SERVING: *Choices/Exchanges: 1½ Carbohydrate; 1 Fat; Calories 150 (from Fat 40); Fat 4.5g (Saturated 0.4g, Trans 0.0g); Cholesterol 0mg; Sodium 100mg; Potassium 160mg; Total Carbohydrate 24g (Dietary Fiber 3g, Sugars 8g); Protein 2g; Phosphorus 80mg.*

Buttermilk Biscuits

INGREDIENTS

2 cups high-fiber flour blend (such as King Arthur High-Fiber Flour Blend)

1 tablespoon baking powder

½ teaspoon baking soda

1 cup low-fat buttermilk

3 tablespoons canola oil

DIRECTIONS

1 Preheat the oven to 425 degrees. Lightly spray two cookie sheets with nonstick cooking spray.

2 In a medium bowl, combine the flour, baking powder, and baking soda. Add the buttermilk and oil; mix with a fork until well blended.

3 Drop the dough by heaping tablespoonfuls onto the cookie sheets, 1½ inches apart. Bake for 10–12 minutes until lightly browned.

PER SERVING: *Choices/Exchanges: 1 Starch; Calories 80 (from Fat 15); Fat 1.5g (Saturated 0.2g, Trans 0.0g); Cholesterol 0mg; Sodium 170mg; Potassium 105mg; Total Carbohydrate 17g (Dietary Fiber 3g, Sugars 1g); Protein 3g; Phosphorus 205mg.*

Corn Muffins

PREP TIME: 10 MIN | COOK TIME: 15 MIN | SERVINGS: 12 | SERVING SIZE: 1 MUFFIN

INGREDIENTS

1 cup yellow cornmeal

½ teaspoon baking soda

½ teaspoon baking powder

¼ teaspoon salt

1 cup low-fat buttermilk

2 egg whites

¼ cup ground flax seeds

1 tablespoon canola oil

½ cup cooked corn kernels

½ cup finely diced red pepper

½ cup finely diced onions, sautéed

DIRECTIONS

1 Preheat the oven to 425 degrees.

2 In a medium bowl, combine the cornmeal, baking soda, baking powder, and salt; mix thoroughly. Stir in the buttermilk, egg whites, flax seeds, and oil; blend well. Mix in the corn, red pepper, and onions. Stir well to combine.

3 Coat the muffin pans with nonstick cooking spray or line with muffin liners. Spoon the batter into the muffin pans, filling the cups ⅔ full. Bake for 10–12 minutes or until the tops are golden brown. Serve warm.

PER SERVING: *Choices/Exchanges: 1 Starch; Calories 90 (from Fat 20); Fat 2.5g (Saturated 0.3g, Trans 0.0g); Cholesterol 0mg; Sodium 150mg; Potassium 115mg; Total Carbohydrate 13g (Dietary Fiber 2g, Sugars 2g); Protein 3g; Phosphorus 70mg.*

Homemade Seasoned Bread Crumbs

INGREDIENTS

One 5-ounce loaf whole-wheat baguette, cut into thin slices, and then into cubes

1 teaspoon dried thyme

1 teaspoon dried oregano

1 teaspoon dried mint

¼ teaspoon paprika

¼ teaspoon salt

¼ teaspoon freshly ground black pepper

DIRECTIONS

1 Preheat the oven to 350 degrees. Place the bread cubes on a baking sheet. Bake for 10–15 minutes or until lightly golden and hard.

2 Allow the bread to cool, and place it in a food processor or blender. Add the remaining ingredients, and process to make crumbs.

PER SERVING: *Choices/Exchanges: ½ Starch; Calories 50 (from Fat 0); Fat 0g (Saturated 0.1g, Trans 0.0g); Cholesterol 0mg; Sodium 160 mg; Potassium 25mg; Total Carbohydrate 9g (Dietary Fiber 1g, Sugars 1g); Protein 2g; Phosphorus 40mg.*

Irish Soda Bread

PREP TIME: ABOUT 5 MIN	COOK TIME: 20 MIN	SERVINGS: 10	SERVING SIZE: 1 SLICE

INGREDIENTS

2 cups high-fiber flour blend (such as King Arthur High-Fiber Flour Blend)

1 teaspoon baking soda

2 tablespoons canola oil

1 tablespoon caraway seeds

¼ cup dried currants or raisins

1 cup low-fat buttermilk

DIRECTIONS

1 Preheat the oven to 375 degrees.

2 In a medium bowl, combine the flour and baking soda. Stir in the oil until the mixture resembles coarse crumbs.

3 Toss in the caraway seeds and currants or raisins. With a fork, mix in the buttermilk until just blended. Turn the dough out onto a lightly floured surface and knead very gently for 20 strokes, just until smooth. Do not overwork the dough.

4 Pat well into a 9-inch pan or shape well on a baking sheet. Make a shallow 4-inch cross in the center of the loaf, and bake for 25–30 minutes until golden. Serve warm.

PER SERVING: *Choices/Exchanges: 1 Starch, ½ Carbohydrate, ½ Fat; Calories 120 (from Fat 30); Fat 3.5g (Saturated 0.3g, Trans 0.0g); Cholesterol 0mg; Sodium 150mg; Potassium 170mg; Total Carbohydrate 23g (Dietary Fiber 5g, Sugars 4g); Protein 3g; Phosphorus 115mg.*

Spoon Bread

INGREDIENTS

2 cups water, divided

1¾ cups yellow cornmeal

½ cup frozen corn kernels, thawed

½ cup ground flaxseeds

2 teaspoons baking powder

1½ teaspoons baking soda

2 cups fat-free milk

2 egg whites

DIRECTIONS

1 In a medium bowl, combine 1 cup of the water with the cornmeal, corn, flaxseeds, baking powder, 1 teaspoon salt (if desired), and baking soda.

2 In a 3-quart saucepan, heat the remaining 1 cup of water to boiling; reduce the heat to low and stir in the cornmeal mixture. Cook the mixture until thick, and remove from the heat.

3 Preheat the oven to 350 degrees. Lightly spray a 2-quart casserole dish with nonstick cooking spray.

4 Add the milk and the egg substitute to the cornmeal mixture, and beat until smooth. Pour into the casserole dish. Bake for 1 hour until set; serve warm.

PER SERVING: *Choices/Exchanges: 1 Starch; Calories 90 (from Fat 15); Fat 1.5g (Saturated 0.2g, Trans 0.0g); Cholesterol 0mg; Sodium 190mg; Potassium 110mg; Total Carbohydrate 16g (Dietary Fiber 2g, Sugars 2g); Protein 3g; Phosphorus 125mg.*

Sweet Potato and Zucchini Bread

PREP TIME: 10 MIN PLUS COOLING TIME	COOK TIME: 1 HR 15 MIN	SERVINGS: 16	SERVING SIZE: 1 SLICE

INGREDIENTS

2 cups high-fiber flour blend (such as King Arthur High Fiber Flour Blend)

¼ teaspoon ground flaxseed

1 teaspoon baking powder

½ teaspoon baking soda

2 teaspoons cinnamon

3 egg whites

1 cup unsweetened applesauce

¼ cup agave nectar

1 teaspoon vanilla extract

1½ cups grated zucchini, unpeeled

1½ cups grated raw sweet potato, peeled

DIRECTIONS

1 Preheat the oven to 350 degrees. Spray a 9-x-5-x-3-inch loaf pan with nonstick cooking spray, and set aside.

2 In a medium bowl, combine the flour, flaxseed, baking powder, baking soda, and cinnamon.

3 In a large bowl, beat together the egg whites, applesauce, agave nectar, and vanilla. Mix in the zucchini and sweet potatoes. Add the flour mixture to the bowl, and mix well.

4 Transfer the batter to the prepared pan; bake for 1 hour and 15 minutes. Cool bread in the pan for 15 minutes. Turn the bread onto a rack, and cool completely. Slice and serve.

PER SERVING: *Choices/Exchanges: 1 Starch, ½ Carbohydrate; Calories 80 (from Fat 0); Fat 0.0g (Saturated 0.0g, Trans 0.0g); Cholesterol 0mg; Sodium 80mg; Potassium 150mg; Total Carbohydrate 20g (Dietary Fiber 3g, Sugars 6g); Protein 3g; Phosphorus 95mg.*

Chapter **15**
Desserts

RECIPES IN THIS CHAPTER

A great dessert can bring a smile to everyone's face. Whether it's a special occasion or just a weeknight, cutting into a pie or cake or biting into a freshly baked cookie is a joyful experience. Living with diabetes doesn't mean you have to miss out on that experience. But because many desserts are high in sugar, carbohydrate, and fat, it's important to look for healthier versions of your favorite dessert recipes.

This chapter offers a wide variety of delicious, diabetes-friendly desserts — from classic cakes, cookies, and cobblers to unique desserts like Cherry Soufflé, Strawberries Romanoff, and Chocolate Fig Pie. You'll also find some basic recipes like the Basic Pie Crust; Low-Calorie, Fat-Free Whipped Cream; and Low-Fat Cream Cheese Frosting that you can use to create healthier versions of your own dessert recipes!

You shouldn't reach for a dessert every night, but it's fine to indulge once in a while. The trick to incorporating the occasional dessert into a diabetes diet is to plan for them. If you'd like to enjoy a slice of pie after dinner, you can make room for it by skipping that starchy side dish or garlic bread on your dinner plate. Just be conscious of portion sizes and make sure you account for any sweet treats in your meal plan.

Maintaining the pleasure of eating is important, so we hope the incredible desserts in this chapter will get you excited about eating well with diabetes and make your life just a little bit sweeter!

Apple Cinnamon Bread Pudding

| PREP TIME: ABOUT 5 MIN | COOK TIME: 1 HR | SERVINGS: 10 | SERVING SIZE: ½ CUP |

INGREDIENTS

9 slices whole-wheat bread, cubed (about 5–6 cups)

2 cups cubed apples (Granny Smith apples work well)

4 cups fat-free milk

1 cup egg substitute

2 teaspoon vanilla

2 teaspoon cinnamon

¼ cup agave nectar

½ cup raisins

DIRECTIONS

1 Preheat the oven to 350 degrees.

2 In a large baking dish, combine the bread and apples.

3 In a bowl, whisk together the milk, egg substitute, vanilla, cinnamon, and agave nectar. Add the raisins. Pour the milk mixture over the bread, and let stand for 15 minutes so the bread can absorb some of the liquid.

4 Bake at 350 degrees for 40–45 minutes, until the bread pudding is set and firm. Cut into squares, and serve warm with whipped topping or low-fat ice cream.

TIP: Serve this pudding warm on those chilly winter nights!

VARY IT! Pears could be substituted for the apples in this recipe. Chopped walnuts also make a great addition.

PER SERVING: Choices/Exchanges: ½ Starch, ½ Fruit, ½ Fat-Free Milk, ½ Carbohydrate; Calories 170 (from Fat 10); Fat 1.0g (Saturated 0.2g, Trans 0.0g); Cholesterol 0mg; Sodium 200mg; Potassium 340mg; Total Carbohydrate 32g (Dietary Fiber 3g, Sugars 19g); Protein 9g, Phosphorus 165mg.

Banana Pineapple Freeze

PREP TIME: ABOUT 5 MIN PLUS CHILLING TIME | SERVINGS: 12 | SERVING SIZE: ½ CUP

INGREDIENTS

2 cups mashed ripe bananas

2 cups unsweetened orange juice

2 tablespoon fresh lemon juice

1 cup unsweetened crushed pineapple, undrained

½ teaspoon ground cinnamon

DIRECTIONS

1 In a food processor, combine all ingredients, and process until smooth and creamy.

2 Pour the mixture into a 9-x-9-x-2-inch baking dish, and freeze overnight or until firm. Serve chilled.

TIP: Try this dessert when you're in the mood for something cool and creamy without all the fat of ice cream. It's especially pretty served in wine or champagne glasses and topped with a sprig of mint.

VARY IT! Mango and guava make great substitutions for the orange juice in this recipe.

PER SERVING: *Choices/Exchanges: 1 Fruit; Calories 60 (from Fat 0); Fat 0.0g (Saturated 0.1g, Trans 0.0g); Cholesterol 0mg; Sodium 0mg; Potassium 240mg; Total Carbohydrate 16g (Dietary Fiber 1g, Sugars 10g); Protein 1g; Phosphorus 15mg.*

Bananas Foster

PREP TIME: ABOUT 5 MIN	COOK TIME: 10 MIN	SERVINGS: 8	SERVING SIZE: 3 SLICES BANANA, ¼ CUP ICE CREAM, AND ⅛ CUP BANANA SAUCE

INGREDIENTS

½ cup unsweetened pineapple juice

¼ teaspoon cinnamon

3 large bananas

1 cup unsweetened sliced pineapple, drained

¼ cup rum

2 cups fat-free, no-sugar-added vanilla ice cream

DIRECTIONS

1 In a medium skillet, combine the pineapple juice and cinnamon.

2 Peel the bananas, and slice in half crosswise; quarter each piece lengthwise.

3 Add the bananas and pineapple slices to the juice mixture, and cook over medium heat until the bananas are soft, basting constantly with juice.

4 Place the rum in a small, long-handled skillet, and heat until warm. Ignite the rum with a long match and quickly pour over the fruit.

5 Arrange the ice cream in a serving dish, spoon the bananas over the ice cream, and serve immediately.

PER SERVING: *Choices/Exchanges: 1 Fruit, 1 Carbohydrate; Calories 120 (from Fat 0); Fat 0.0g (Saturated 0.1g, Trans 0.0g); Cholesterol 0mg; Sodium 35mg; Potassium 320mg; Total Carbohydrate 27g (Dietary Fiber 4g, Sugars 13g); Protein 3g; Phosphorus 40mg.*

Classic Crêpes

PREP TIME: ABOUT 5 MIN PLUS CHILLING TIME	COOK TIME: 10 MIN	SERVINGS: 10	SERVING SIZE: TWO 6-INCH CRÊPES

INGREDIENTS

¾ cup egg substitute

1⅓ cups buckwheat flour

½ teaspoon salt

1½ cups fat-free milk

2 teaspoons canola oil

DIRECTIONS

1 In a food processor or blender, combine all ingredients. Process for 30 seconds, scraping down the sides of the container. Continue to process until the mixture is smooth; refrigerate for 1 hour.

2 Coat the bottom of a 6-inch crêpe pan or small skillet with nonstick cooking spray. Place the pan over medium heat until hot but not smoking.

3 Pour 2 tablespoons of the batter into the pan, and quickly tilt it in all directions so the batter covers the pan in a thin film. Cook for about 1 minute, lifting the edge of the crêpe to test for doneness. The crêpe is ready to be flipped when it can be shaken loose from the pan.

4 Flip the crêpe, and continue to cook for 30 seconds on the other side. (This side usually has brownish spots on it, so place the filling on this side.)

5 Stack the cooked crêpes between layers of wax paper to avoid sticking, and repeat the process with the remaining batter.

VARY IT! Any filling is great stuffed into these basic crêpes, depending on whether you're serving hearty main entrees or spectacular desserts!

PER SERVING: *Choices/Exchanges: 1 Starch; Calories 80 (from Fat 15); Fat 1.5g (Saturated 0.2g, Trans 0.0g); Cholesterol 0mg; Sodium 170mg; Potassium 180mg; Total Carbohydrate 13g (Dietary Fiber 2g, Sugars 2g); Protein 5g; Phosphorus 95mg.*

Carrot Cake

PREP TIME: ABOUT 10 MIN	COOK TIME: 40 MIN	SERVINGS: 16	SERVING SIZE: 1 SLICE

INGREDIENTS

½ cup canola oil

½ cup unsweetened applesauce

2 tablespoons granulated sugar substitute (such as stevia)

1 cup egg substitute

½ cup water

2 cups whole-wheat flour

1 teaspoon baking powder

1 teaspoon baking soda

2 teaspoons cinnamon

¼ teaspoon nutmeg

½ teaspoon salt

¾ cup chopped pecans

3 cups grated carrots

DIRECTIONS

1 Preheat the oven to 350 degrees.

2 In a large mixing bowl, beat together the oil, applesauce, sugar substitute, and egg substitute until well blended.

3 Add the water, flour, baking powder, baking soda, cinnamon, and nutmeg, and mix well. Stir in the pecans and carrots.

4 Coat a 3-quart tube pan with nonstick cooking spray. Pour in the batter and bake at 350 degrees for 35–40 minutes or until a toothpick inserted in the cake comes out clean.

5 Let the cake cool 10 minutes in the pan, and then invert the cake onto a plate and let it cool completely. If you like, frost with Low-Fat Cream Cheese Frosting (see the recipe later in this chapter).

VARY IT! Almond flour can be swapped out for regular flour for a gluten-free variation. Or you can substitute zucchini for the carrots for a moist zucchini cake.

PER SERVING: Choices/Exchanges: 1 Carbohydrate, 2 Fat; Calories 170 (from Fat 100); Fat 11.0g (Saturated 0.9g, Trans 0.0g); Cholesterol 0mg; Sodium 150mg; Potassium 180mg; Total Carbohydrate 15g (Dietary Fiber 3g, Sugars 2g); Protein 4g; Phosphorus 105mg.

Cherry Almond Cobbler

INGREDIENTS

2 cups water-packed sour cherries

¼ teaspoon fresh lemon juice

⅛ teaspoon almond extract

½ cup almond flour, sifted

⅛ teaspoon salt

¼ cup flaxseeds

¾ teaspoon baking powder

1 tablespoon canola oil

¼ cup egg substitute

2 tablespoons fat-free milk

¼ cup granulated sugar substitute (such as stevia)

DIRECTIONS

1 Preheat the oven to 425 degrees. Drain the cherries, reserving ⅔ cup of liquid, and place the cherries in a shallow 9-inch glass or porcelain cake pan.

2 In a small mixing bowl, combine the lemon juice, almond extract, and drained cherry liquid; mix well. Spoon over the cherries.

3 In a mixing bowl, combine the almond flour, flaxseeds, and baking powder. Mix thoroughly. Stir in the oil, egg substitute, milk, and sugar substitute, mixing well.

4 Spoon the mixture over the cherries, and bake at 425 degrees for 25–30 minutes or until the crust is golden brown.

VARY IT! Blueberries or a mixture of berries can be swapped out for the cherries in this recipe.

PER SERVING: *Choices/Exchanges: ½ Fruit, ½ Carbohydrate, 1 Lean Protein, 2½ Fat; Calories 230 (from Fat 140); Fat 15.0g (Saturated 1.2g, Trans 0.0g); Cholesterol 0mg; Sodium 115mg; Potassium 340mg; Total Carbohydrate 19g (Dietary Fiber 6g, Sugars 11g); Protein 8g; Phosphorus 240mg.*

Cherry Soufflé

PREP TIME: ABOUT 5 MIN PLUS CHILLING TIME	COOK TIME: 15 MIN	SERVINGS: 4	SERVING SIZE: ½ CUP

INGREDIENTS

⅓ cup water

½ package unflavored gelatin

1 cup water-packed sour cherries, drained and chopped, divided

1 tablespoon fresh lemon juice

2 tablespoons granulated sugar substitute (such as stevia)

2 large egg whites, beaten to soft peaks

½ cup slivered almonds

1 cup prepared Low-Calorie, Fat-Free Whipped Cream (see recipe later in this chapter)

DIRECTIONS

1 In a medium saucepan, combine the water and gelatin; allow to soften for 10–15 minutes. Add ½ cup of the cherries, lemon juice, and sugar substitute; bring to a boil.

2 Remove from the heat, and let cool; refrigerate until thick and syrupy.

3 Fold in the remaining cherries, beaten egg whites, almonds, and whipped cream. Spoon into a soufflé dish, and refrigerate until set.

PER SERVING: *Choices/Exchanges: 1 Carbohydrate, 1 Lean Protein, 1 Fat; Calories 160 (from Fat 70); Fat 8.0g (Saturated 0.6g, Trans 0.0g); Cholesterol 0mg; Sodium 85mg; Potassium 340mg; Total Carbohydrate 15g (Dietary Fiber 2g, Sugars 11g); Protein 10g; Phosphorus 160mg.*

Chocolate Chip and Cranberry Cookies

PREP TIME: ABOUT 5 MIN PLUS CHILLING TIME	COOK TIME: 10 MIN	SERVINGS: 15	SERVING SIZE: 2 COOKIES

INGREDIENTS

¼ cup canola oil

¼ cup granulated sugar substitute (such as stevia)

1 egg white

1 teaspoon vanilla

1 cup almond flour

¼ teaspoon baking soda

¼ teaspoon salt

4 tablespoons semisweet chocolate mini morsels

½ cup dried cranberries

½ cup chopped walnuts

DIRECTIONS

1 Preheat the oven to 375 degrees.

2 In a medium bowl, cream the oil and sugar substitute, Beat in the egg white and vanilla; mix thoroughly.

3 In a sifter, combine the flour, baking soda, and salt. Sift the dry ingredients into the creamed mixture, and mix well. Stir in the chocolate mini morsels, cranberries, and walnuts.

4 Lightly spray cookie sheets with nonstick cooking spray. Drop teaspoonfuls of dough onto the cookie sheet. Place in the freezer for 10 minutes to chill.

5 Bake at 375 degrees for 8–10 minutes. Remove the cookies from the oven, and cool them on racks.

PER SERVING: *Choices/Exchanges: ½ Carbohydrate, 2 Fat; Calories 140 (from Fat 100); Fat 11.0g (Saturated 1.5g, Trans 0.0g); Cholesterol 0mg; Sodium 65mg; Potassium 90mg; Total Carbohydrate 8g (Dietary Fiber 2g, Sugars 5g); Protein 3g; Phosphorus 55mg.*

Chocolate Cupcakes

PREP TIME: ABOUT 10 MIN	COOK TIME: 20 MIN	SERVINGS: 12	SERVING SIZE: 1 CUPCAKE

INGREDIENTS

3 tablespoons canola oil

¼ cup agave nectar

¼ cup egg whites

1 teaspoon vanilla

1 teaspoon cold espresso or strong coffee

½ cup fat-free milk

1¼ cups quinoa flour

¼ cup ground walnuts

6 tablespoons cocoa powder

2 teaspoons baking powder

¼ teaspoon baking soda

DIRECTIONS

1 Preheat the oven to 375 degrees.

2 In a medium bowl, beat the oil with the agave nectar, egg whites, vanilla, espresso, and milk.

3 In a separate bowl, combine the quinoa flour, walnuts, cocoa powder, baking powder, and baking soda. Add to the creamed mixture, and mix until smooth.

4 Spoon the batter into paper–lined muffin tins, and bake at 375 degrees for 20 minutes. Remove from the oven and let cool.

TIP: Try frosting these with Low-Fat Cream Cheese Frosting (see the recipe later in this chapter).

PER SERVING: *Choices/Exchanges: ½ Starch, ½ Carbohydrate, 1 Fat; Calories 120 (from Fat 50); Fat 6.0g (Saturated 0.7g, Trans 0.0g); Cholesterol 0mg; Sodium 105mg; Potassium 160mg; Total Carbohydrate 15g (Dietary Fiber 2g, Sugars 5g); Protein 3g; Phosphorus 160mg.*

Chocolate Fig Pie

PREP TIME: ABOUT 10 MIN PLUS CHILLING TIME | COOK TIME: 20 MIN | SERVINGS: 9 | SERVING SIZE: 1 SLICE

INGREDIENTS

1 package unflavored gelatin

1 cup fat-free milk

2 eggs, separated

2 tablespoons agave nectar

¼ cup cocoa

1 teaspoon vanilla extract

1 cup dried figs, trimmed and quartered

2 cups fat-free whipped topping

1 prepared Basic Pie Crust, baked (see recipe later in this chapter)

DIRECTIONS

1 In a large saucepan, combine the gelatin, milk, egg yolks, agave, and cocoa. Cook over medium heat until completely blended and slightly thickened.

2 Remove from the heat, stir in the vanilla extract, and refrigerate the mixture until partially set.

3 In a small bowl, beat the egg whites until stiff peaks form. Fold into the cooled chocolate mixture. Fold in the figs.

4 Layer the chocolate mixture and whipped topping in the pie shell, ending with whipped topping. Refrigerate for 2–3 hours or until firm. Cut into 9 slices and enjoy.

VARY IT! Omit the cocoa for a Vanilla Fig Pie.

PER SERVING: Choices/Exchanges: 2 Carbohydrate, 1 Fat; Calories 200 (from Fat 50); Fat 6.0g (Saturated 0.9g, Trans 0.0g); Cholesterol 40mg; Sodium 55mg; Potassium 240mg; Total Carbohydrate 31g (Dietary Fiber 3g, Sugars 15g); Protein 5g; Phosphorus 100mg.

Crêpes Suzette

INGREDIENTS

2 cups unsweetened orange juice

2 tablespoons cornstarch

1 tablespoon orange zest

2 medium oranges, peeled and sectioned

16 Classic Crêpes (see recipe earlier in this chapter)

¼ cup orange liqueur (such as Grand Marnier)

DIRECTIONS

1 In a large skillet, combine the orange juice, cornstarch, and orange zest. Bring the mixture to a boil over medium heat. Boil for 1–2 minutes, stirring occasionally.

2 Add the orange sections and remove from the heat. Allow the mixture to cool slightly.

3 Dip both sides of the crêpes in the sauce; fold in quarters. Arrange the crêpes in the skillet in the remaining sauce; heat completely over low heat.

4 Heat (do not boil!) the orange liqueur in a saucepan over medium heat, then carefully ignite it with a long match, and pour over the crêpes. Serve when the flame subsides.

PER SERVING: *Choices/Exchanges: 1 Starch, 1 Fruit; Calories 150 (from Fat 15); Fat 1.5g (Saturated 0.2g, Trans 0.0g); Cholesterol 0mg; Sodium 170mg; Potassium 370mg; Total Carbohydrate 28g (Dietary Fiber 3g, Sugars 12g); Protein 6g; Phosphorus 110mg.*

Crumb Pie Shell

PREP TIME: ABOUT 10 MIN | COOK TIME: 10 MIN | SERVINGS: 10 | SERVING SIZE: ONE 1-INCH SLICE

INGREDIENTS

1¼ cups finely crumbled high-fiber bran crisp breads (such as Fiber Rich+ Bran Crisp Breads)

2 tablespoons canola oil

1 tablespoon water

⅛ teaspoon cinnamon

DIRECTIONS

1 Preheat the oven to 325 degrees. In a medium mixing bowl, combine all the ingredients, mixing thoroughly.

2 Spread the mixture evenly into a 10-inch pie pan. Press the mixture firmly onto the sides and bottom of the pan.

3 Bake the pie shell for 8–10 minutes. You can refrigerate it after baking until ready to use.

TIP: You can use this basic crumb pie shell with almost any filling.

PER SERVING: *Choices/Exchanges: ½ Starch; ½ Fat; Calories 45 (from Fat 25); Fat 3.0g (Saturated 0.2g, Trans 0.0g); Cholesterol 0mg; Sodium 0mg; Potassium 20mg; Total Carbohydrate 6g (Dietary Fiber 3g, Sugars 0g); Protein 1g; Phosphorus 20mg.*

Fresh Apple Pie

PREP TIME: ABOUT 10 MIN	COOK TIME: 40 MIN	SERVINGS: 9	SERVING SIZE: ONE 1-INCH SLICE

INGREDIENTS

10 medium baking apples (Rome apples work well), peeled, cored, and sliced (3 pounds total)

2 teaspoons fresh lemon juice

1 prepared Basic Pie Crust, unbaked (see recipe later in this chapter)

2 tablespoons granulated sugar substitute (such as stevia)

1 tablespoon flour

1 teaspoon ground cinnamon

½ cup walnuts, chopped

½ teaspoon ground nutmeg

DIRECTIONS

1 Preheat the oven to 425 degrees.

2 Place the sliced apples in a large bowl, sprinkle with lemon juice, and toss to coat. Arrange the apples in the pie shell.

3 In a small bowl, combine the sugar substitute, flour, cinnamon, walnuts, and nutmeg; mix well. Sprinkle the mixture over the apples.

4 Cover the edges of the crust with aluminum foil, so they don't burn. Bake the pie at 425 degrees for 35–40 minutes or until the crust is golden brown. Remove from the oven, and cool slightly before serving.

VARY IT! You can substitute peaches or berries for the apples in this delicious homemade pie.

PER SERVING: *Choices/Exchanges: ½ Starch, 1 Fruit, ½ Carbohydrate; 1½ Fat; Calories 190 (from Fat 80); Fat 9.0g (Saturated 0.8g, Trans 0.0g); Cholesterol 0mg; Sodium 15mg; Potassium 160mg; Total Carbohydrate 28g (Dietary Fiber 2g; Sugars 14g); Protein 2g; Phosphorus 50mg.*

Basic Pie Crust

PREP TIME: ABOUT 10 MIN PLUS CHILLING TIME	COOK TIME: 40 MIN	SERVINGS: 9	SERVING SIZE: ONE 1-INCH SLICE

INGREDIENTS

¾ cup cake flour

½ teaspoon sugar

¹⁄₁₆ teaspoon salt

3 tablespoons canola oil, frozen for 15 minutes

½ teaspoon white vinegar

2 tablespoons ice water

DIRECTIONS

1 In a medium bowl, combine the flour, sugar, and salt. Stir in the oil and mix until the mixture is the size of small peas.

2 Add the vinegar and ice water and mix with a fork until the dough starts to hold together. Gather into a ball, wrap, and refrigerate at least 30 minutes before rolling out.

3 Roll out the pie crust to fit an 8- or 9-inch pie dish. Lay the rolled dough in the pan without stretching it, and crimp the edges.

4 If the recipe requires a baked pie crust, preheat the oven to 425 degrees. Prick the crust with a fork, and lay a piece of parchment or wax paper in the pie shell. Pour in enough dried beans to cover the bottom (this prevents the crust from bubbling up while baking). Bake for 8 minutes or until golden brown.

PER SERVING: *Choices/Exchanges: ½ Starch, 1 Fat; Calories 80 (from Fat 45); Fat 5.0g (Saturated 0.4g, Trans 0.0g); Cholesterol 0mg; Sodium 15mg; Potassium 10mg; Total Carbohydrate 9g (Dietary Fiber 0g, Sugars 0g); Protein 1g; Phosphorus 10mg.*

Low-Calorie, Fat-Free Whipped Cream

PREP TIME: ABOUT 5 MIN	COOK TIME: 5 MIN	SERVINGS: 8	SERVING SIZE: 2 TABLESPOONS

INGREDIENTS

2 tablespoons water

1 teaspoon unflavored gelatin

½ cup fat-free powdered milk

1 teaspoon vanilla extract

1 cup ice water

½ teaspoon agave nectar

DIRECTIONS

1 In a small skillet, add the water; sprinkle gelatin on top.

2 After the gelatin has soaked in, stir over low heat until clear; cool. In a large mixing bowl, combine the milk, vanilla, ice water, and agave nectar; mix well.

3 Add the gelatin mixture, and whip until fluffy with a wire whisk or electric beaters. Refrigerate the whipped cream until ready to use.

PER SERVING: *Choices/Exchanges: Free Food; Calories 20 (from Fat 0); Fat 0.0g (Saturated 0.0g, Trans 0.0g); Cholesterol 0mg; Sodium 25mg; Potassium 75mg; Total Carbohydrate 3g (Dietary Fiber 0g, Sugars 3g); Protein 2g; Phosphorus 40mg.*

Low-Fat Cream Cheese Frosting

PREP TIME: ABOUT 5 MIN | **SERVINGS: 48** | **SERVING SIZE: 2 TABLESPOONS**

INGREDIENTS

3 cups fat-free ricotta cheese

1⅓ cups plain fat-free yogurt, strained overnight in cheesecloth over a bowl set in the refrigerator

2 cups low-fat cottage cheese

⅓ cup fructose

3 tablespoons evaporated fat-free milk

DIRECTIONS

1 In a large bowl, combine all the ingredients; beat well with electric beaters until slightly stiff.

2 Place frosting in a covered container, and refrigerate until ready to use (this frosting can be refrigerated for up to 1 week).

PER SERVING: *Choices/Exchanges: Free Food; Calories 25 (from Fat 0); Fat 0.0g (Saturated 0.1g, Trans 0.0g); Cholesterol 5mg; Sodium 55mg; Potassium 40mg; Total Carbohydrate 3g (Dietary Fiber 0g, Sugars 2g); Protein 4g; Phosphorus 50mg.*

Oatmeal Raisin Cookies

PREP TIME: ABOUT 5 MIN	COOK TIME: 15 MIN	SERVINGS: 16	SERVING SIZE: 3 COOKIES

INGREDIENTS

3 cups rolled oats

1 cup whole-wheat flour

1 teaspoon baking soda

2 teaspoons cinnamon

½ cup raisins

¼ cup unsweetened applesauce

¼ cup agave nectar

½ cup egg substitute

½ cup plain fat-free yogurt

1 teaspoon vanilla

DIRECTIONS

1 Preheat the oven to 350 degrees.

2 In a medium bowl, combine the oats, flour, baking soda, cinnamon, and raisins.

3 In a large bowl, beat the applesauce, agave nectar, egg substitute, yogurt, and vanilla until creamy. Slowly add the dry ingredients, and mix together.

4 Spray cookie sheets with nonstick cooking spray, and drop by teaspoonfuls onto the cookie sheets. Bake for 12–15 minutes at 350 degrees; transfer to racks, and cool.

PER SERVING: *Choices/Exchanges: 1 Starch, ½ Carbohydrate; Calories 120 (from Fat 10); Fat 1.0g (Saturated 0.2g, Trans 0.0g); Cholesterol 0mg; Sodium 100mg; Potassium 150mg; Total Carbohydrate 25g (Dietary Fiber 3g, Sugars 7g); Protein 4g; Phosphorus 105mg.*

Peach Crumb Cobbler

PREP TIME: ABOUT 5 MIN	COOK TIME: 30 MIN	SERVINGS: 3	SERVING SIZE: ⅓ COBBLER

INGREDIENTS

2 cups fresh peaches, sliced

⅓ cup graham cracker crumbs

½ teaspoon ground cinnamon

¼ teaspoon nutmeg

2 teaspoons canola oil

DIRECTIONS

1 Preheat the oven to 350 degrees.

2 Place the sliced peaches in the bottom of an 8-x-8-x-2-inch baking pan.

3 In a small mixing bowl, combine the graham cracker crumbs, cinnamon, and nutmeg; mix well.

4 Gradually blend in the oil, and sprinkle the mixture over the peaches. Bake uncovered at 350 degrees for 25–30 minutes. Remove from the oven, and let cool slightly before serving.

VARY IT! You can substitute pears, apples, or berries for the peaches in this tasty cobbler.

PER SERVING: *Choices/Exchanges: ½ Starch, ½ Fruit, 1 Fat; Calories 110 (from Fat 40); Fat 4.5g (Saturated 0.4g, Trans 0.0g); Cholesterol 0mg; Sodium 55mg; Potassium 210mg; Total Carbohydrate 17g (Dietary Fiber 2g, Sugars 12g); Protein 2g; Phosphorus 30mg.*

Peach Shortcake

PREP TIME: ABOUT 10 MIN	COOK TIME: 30 MIN	SERVINGS: 8	SERVING SIZE: ½ CUP

INGREDIENTS

2½ cups sliced fresh peaches

½ cup slivered almonds

1½ tablespoons plus 1 teaspoon granulated sugar substitute (such as stevia), divided

½ teaspoon almond extract

½ teaspoon cinnamon

1 cup whole-wheat flour

2 teaspoons baking powder

2 tablespoons canola oil

¼ cup egg substitute

¼ cup fat-free milk

DIRECTIONS

1 Preheat the oven to 400 degrees.

2 Lightly spray an 8-x-8-x-2-inch baking pan with nonstick cooking spray. Arrange the peaches and almonds in the bottom of the dish.

3 In a small bowl, mix together 1 teaspoon of the sugar substitute, the almond extract, and the cinnamon; sprinkle over the peaches, and set aside.

4 In a medium bowl, combine the flour, baking powder, and the remaining 1½ tablespoons of sugar substitute; mix well.

5 Add the oil, egg substitute, and milk to the dry ingredients; mix until smooth. Spread evenly over the peaches, and bake for 25–30 minutes or until the top is golden brown. Remove from the oven, invert onto a serving plate, and serve.

PER SERVING: *Choices/Exchanges: ½ Starch, ½ Fruit, 1½ Fat; Calories 150 (from Fat 70); Fat 8.0g (Saturated 0.6g, Trans 0.0g); Cholesterol 0mg; Sodium 110mg; Potassium 230mg; Total Carbohydrate 18g (Dietary Fiber 3g, Sugars 5g); Protein 5g; Phosphorus 220mg.*

Pineapple Pear Medley

PREP TIME: ABOUT 10 MIN PLUS CHILLING TIME	COOK TIME: 10 MIN	SERVINGS: 12	SERVING SIZE: ½ CUP

INGREDIENTS

1 large orange

15 ounces canned unsweetened pineapple chunks, undrained

32 ounces canned unsweetened pear halves, drained

16 ounces canned unsweetened apricot halves, drained

6 whole cloves

2 cinnamon sticks

DIRECTIONS

1 Peel the orange, and reserve the rind. Divide the orange into sections, and remove the membrane.

2 Drain the pineapple, reserve the juice, and set aside.

3 In a large bowl, combine the orange sections, pineapple, pears, and apricots. Toss, and set aside.

4 In a small saucepan over medium heat, combine the orange rind, pineapple juice, cloves, and cinnamon. Let simmer for 5–10 minutes; then strain the juices, and pour over the fruit.

5 Cover, and refrigerate for at least 2–3 hours. Toss before serving.

PER SERVING: *Choices/Exchanges: 1 Fruit; Calories 60 (from Fat 0); Fat 0.0g (Saturated 0.0g, Trans 0.0g); Cholesterol 0mg; Sodium 0mg; Potassium 150mg; Total Carbohydrate 16g (Dietary Fiber 2g, Sugars 13g); Protein 1g; Phosphorus 15mg.*

Baked Pumpkin Pudding

PREP TIME: ABOUT 5 MIN | COOK TIME: 20 MIN | SERVINGS: 4 | SERVING SIZE: ½ CUP

INGREDIENTS

1½ cups mashed pumpkin

1 egg

2½ tablespoons agave nectar

½ teaspoon vanilla extract

1 teaspoon pumpkin pie spice

¼ cup slivered almonds

¼ cup raisins

DIRECTIONS

1 Preheat the oven to 350 degrees.

2 In a large bowl, combine the pumpkin, egg, agave nectar, vanilla, and pumpkin pie spice, and mix well. Stir in the almonds and raisins, leaving a few for garnish.

3 Spoon the mixture into 4 ramekins, and garnish with the remaining almonds and raisins.

4 Bake at 350 degrees for approximately 20 minutes, or until golden on top.

5 Serve warm or at room temperature. Top with Low-Calorie, Fat-Free Whipped Cream if desired (see the recipe earlier in this chapter).

PER SERVING: *Choices/Exchanges: 2 Carbohydrate, 1 Fat; Calories 160 (from Fat 45); Fat 5.0g (Saturated 0.8g, Trans 0.0g); Cholesterol 45mg; Sodium 25mg; Potassium 330mg; Total Carbohydrate 26g (Dietary Fiber 4g, Sugars 18g); Protein 4g; Phosphorus 100mg.*

Sponge Cake

PREP TIME: 15 MIN | **COOK TIME: 1 HR** | **SERVINGS: 12** | **SERVING SIZE: 1 SLICE**

INGREDIENTS

1 cup fresh berries, rinsed

2 tablespoons balsamic vinegar

2 tablespoons agave nectar

4 large eggs, separated

¼ cup granulated sugar substitute (such as stevia)

½ cup hot water

1½ teaspoons vanilla extract

1½ cups almond flour, sifted

¼ teaspoon salt

¼ teaspoon baking powder

DIRECTIONS

1 Preheat the oven to 325 degrees.

2 In a medium bowl, combine the berries with the balsamic vinegar and agave nectar. Mix well to combine; cover, and set aside to steep.

3 In another medium bowl, beat the egg yolks and sugar substitute until thick and lemon-colored. Add the hot water and vanilla, and continue beating for 3 more minutes.

4 In a large bowl, combine the flour, salt, and baking powder; add to the egg yolk mixture.

5 In a small bowl, beat the egg whites until stiff and fold into the egg yolk mixture. Spoon the batter into an ungreased 9-inch tube pan, and bake at 325 degrees for 50–60 minutes or until a toothpick inserted comes out clean.

6 Remove the cake from the oven, and invert it onto a plate. Allow the cake to sit inverted in its pan for at least 1 hour. Remove the pan and let the cake cool completely. Garnish with fresh berry mixture.

VARY IT! A good ratio of berries is 1/3 cup each of blueberries, strawberries, and raspberries, but you can use any kind of berries you'd like.

PER SERVING: *Choices/Exchanges: ½ Carbohydrate, 2 Fat; Calories 130 (from Fat 80); Fat 9.0g (Saturated 1.1g, Trans 0.0g); Cholesterol 60mg; Sodium 85mg; Potassium 140mg; Total Carbohydrate 8g (Dietary Fiber 2g, Sugars 4g); Protein 5g; Phosphorus 110mg.*

Strawberries Romanoff

PREP TIME: ABOUT 5 MIN | SERVINGS: 4 | SERVING SIZE: ¾ CUP

INGREDIENTS

2 cups fresh strawberries, hulled

1 cup low-fat frozen Greek yogurt

Juice and zest of 1 orange

½ cup prepared Low-Calorie, Fat-Free Whipped Cream (see recipe earlier in chapter)

½ cup peeled, unsalted pistachios, finely chopped

DIRECTIONS

1 Divide the strawberries evenly between 4 serving dishes, and refrigerate.

2 Just before serving, fold the frozen yogurt, orange juice and zest, and whipped cream together in a medium bowl. Spoon evenly over the chilled strawberries, top with pistachios, and serve.

PER SERVING: *Choices/Exchanges: ½ Fat-Free Milk, 1½ Carbohydrate, 1 Fat; Calories 200 (from Fat 70); Fat 8.0g (Saturated 1.3g, Trans 0.0g); Cholesterol 8mg; Sodium 60mg; Potassium 480mg; Total Carbohydrate 26g (Dietary Fiber 3g, Sugars 17g); Protein 8g; Phosphorus 175mg.*

Walnut Macaroons

PREP TIME: ABOUT 5 MIN PLUS CHILLING TIME	COOK TIME: 15 MIN	SERVINGS: 14	SERVING SIZE: 3 COOKIES

INGREDIENTS

2 cups quick-cooking oats

¼ cup dried organic unsweetened coconut

2 tablespoons granulated sugar substitute (such as stevia)

2 teaspoons vanilla extract

½ cup canola oil

¼ cup egg whites, beaten until stiff

½ cup finely chopped walnuts

DIRECTIONS

1 In a medium bowl, combine the oats, coconut, sugar substitute, vanilla, and oil; mix thoroughly. Cover, and refrigerate overnight.

2 Preheat the oven to 350 degrees. Carefully fold the egg whites and walnuts into the mixture; blend thoroughly.

3 Pack the cookie mixture into a teaspoon, level, and push out onto ungreased cookie sheets.

4 Bake the cookies at 350 degrees for 15 minutes or until the tops are golden brown. Transfer the cookies to racks, and cool.

PER SERVING: *Choices/Exchanges: ½ Starch, 2½ Fat; Calories 150 (from Fat 110); Fat 12.0g (Saturated 1.3g, Trans 0.0g); Cholesterol 0mg; Sodium 10mg; Potassium 75mg; Total Carbohydrate 9g (Dietary Fiber 2g, Sugars 0g); Protein 3g; Phosphorus 65mg.*

4

Planning Your Meals

Discover the ins and outs of diabetes meal planning and prepare to meet with a dietitian.

Practice portion control with the Plate Method and other techniques.

Find out which foods contain carbohydrate and develop your carbohydrate-counting skills.

Navigate the food lists for people with diabetes.

Explore eating patterns for people with diabetes and consider fine-tuning your meal plan with the glycemic index.

Chapter **16**

A Little Planning Goes a Long Way

I f you've recently been diagnosed with diabetes, you probably hear the term *meal plan* a lot from your diabetes care team. If you're not familiar with the term, don't worry! We're here to help. Planning your meals is one of the best ways to set yourself up for success when it comes to eating healthy with diabetes.

It's a good idea to have a general understanding of macronutrients (carbohydrate, protein, and fat) when you're developing a diabetes meal plan. Your healthcare provider may have already discussed with you the importance of carbohydrate in diabetes management, but we review the basics of carbohydrate and the other macronutrients — protein and fat — in this chapter. Then we get you started with the first step of effective meal planning: meeting with a dietitian. Finally, we give you an overview of a variety of different meal-planning approaches.

Introducing the Idea of Meal Planning

So, what is a meal plan exactly? For people with diabetes, a *meal plan* is simply a guide that tells you how much and what kinds of foods to eat at meals to keep your body healthy and keep your blood glucose in check. An effective meal plan should take into account your schedule, eating habits, and food preferences. A meal plan can be very simple or a little more complex, depending on your individual needs and diabetes goals. And a meal plan should change over time to adapt to changes in your weight, medications, physical activity level, and diabetes goals.

Common goals that people set when creating a meal plan include the following:

>> Improving blood glucose levels

>> Improving blood pressure and cholesterol levels

>> Losing or maintaining weight

>> Preventing or treating particular diabetes complications

>> Maintaining the joy of eating

You may not share all these goals, but it's important to determine — with the help of your healthcare provider — what diabetes goals you want your meal plan to address. When you understand these goals, it's time to create your meal plan! (We introduce different types of meal plans at the end of this chapter and go into more details about them in the rest of Part 4.)

Defining Macronutrients

Every meal plan is made up of three main components: carbohydrate, protein, and fat — the *macronutrients.* All the foods we eat are made up of some combination of these three nutrients; some foods may have only one nutrient, while other foods may have all three.

REMEMBER

The human body needs all three of these macronutrients to function properly, so you should try to eat a variety of foods to ensure that you get all these different nutrients.

Your healthcare provider or dietitian may help you plan a certain range of grams of carbohydrate, protein, and/or fat to eat each day as part of the meal planning process.

The following sections explain how each macronutrient affects your body and identify some foods choices that represent each nutrient.

Note: The American Diabetes Association doesn't have recommendations regarding the amount of carbohydrate, protein, and fat that people with type 2 diabetes should eat each day. Discuss your personal dietary needs with your healthcare provider or dietitian.

Carbohydrate: Converts into glucose

Carbohydrate is an important nutrient for people with diabetes because it's the nutrient directly responsible for raising your blood glucose levels after eating. During digestion, your body breaks carbohydrate down into glucose, which then enters your bloodstream and causes your blood glucose levels to climb. Therefore, you'll need to consider how you're going to choose carbohydrate foods and manage your carbohydrate intake when building your meal plan. But remember, your body needs some carbohydrate; it fuels your body. So, don't try to remove all carbohydrate from your diet.

Foods that contain carbohydrate include fruits, vegetables, beans, whole grains, breads and crackers, milk and yogurt, and other starchy or sugary foods and drinks. When choosing carbohydrate foods, look for nutrient- and fiber-rich options, and try to limit or avoid processed and sugary sources of carbohydrate such as white breads, white pastas, sugary desserts, and regular sodas.

Protein: Builds strong bodies

Protein is essential for a healthy body. Among other functions, this nutrient helps your body build new tissues and muscles. Foods that are high in protein include poultry, seafood, red meats, dairy products, and even plant-based proteins such as beans, lentils, peas, and soy products. When choosing protein, it's best to stick to lean poultry, fish, and plant-based proteins for most of your meals. Limit your intake of red meats, and avoid high-fat and highly processed sources of protein, such as bacon and sausage, that are high in saturated fat and sodium and add to your risk of heart disease.

Fat: Healthy types are helpful

Most people think fat is harmful for your body. But, as with carbohydrate and protein, your body actually needs a certain amount of fat to stay healthy. However, the body only needs a small amount of fat to function properly. Many people have way too much fat in their diets. Moderation is important when it comes to fat because certain kinds of fat and eating too much fat can increase your risk for cardiovascular complications such as heart disease, heart attack, and stroke. And overindulging in fat can increase your weight.

Some fats are better than others. Saturated fats and trans fats can raise your blood cholesterol levels, so it's a good idea to limit these fats in your meal plan. You'll find these types of harmful fats in butter, stick margarines, cream, cheese, high-fat meats, full-fat dairy products, and certain oils like palm and coconut oils. But there are some healthy fats that can actually have positive effects on your heart health by reducing bad cholesterol levels and preventing clogging in the arteries. These healthy fats — monounsaturated and polyunsaturated fats and omega-3 fatty acids — can be found in avocados, nuts and seeds, many plant oils, and (for omega-3 fatty acids) fish such as albacore tuna, herring, mackerel, rainbow trout, salmon, and sardines. For more information on which foods contain these healthy fats, see Chapter 1.

Healthy fats still need to be enjoyed in moderation, but you can help protect your heart from the effects of saturated and trans fats by replacing the sources of these unhealthy fats with sources of heathy fats. Work with your healthcare provider or dietitian to come up with a personalized strategy for including healthy fats in your meal plan.

First Things First: Meeting with a Dietitian

Many people are surprised to find out that there is no one meal plan or "diabetes diet" that is recommended for all people with diabetes. Your meal plan should be individualized for you. If you've just been diagnosed with diabetes, you'll want to meet with a registered dietitian (RD) or registered dietitian nutritionist (RDN) to develop your personalized meal plan. If you don't have a dietitian, your doctor can give you a referral. You might think you can make a meal plan on your own, but the help of an RD or RDN will make the process so much easier. He or she can answer any questions you have about healthy eating with diabetes.

TECHNICAL
STUFF

A *registered dietitian* (RD) or *registered dietitian nutritionist* (RDN) is a person who is professionally trained to educate people on food, nutrition, and weight management. Some dietitians are also *certified diabetes educators* (CDEs), which means they're specifically trained to work with people with diabetes on all topics related to diabetes management. A CDE can be an excellent resource for you as you begin your journey with diabetes. Your dietitian doesn't have to be a CDE, but finding a dietitian who has experience with diabetes management and nutrition will be helpful.

Your dietitian will work with you to create a meal plan that's best for *you*. This means that he or she will help you

>> Select a meal planning approach that fits your lifestyle, diabetes goals, and eating habits.

>> Determine how many calories and grams or servings of carbohydrate, protein, and fat you should aim to eat each day to meet your diabetes goals.

>> Figure out when, how often, and how much you need to eat.

Is eating three square meals a day right for you? Or will you need a snack or two between meals? Will counting calories and carbohydrates be effective for you? Or should you focus more on portion-control techniques? Your dietitian can help you with these questions and many more.

The meal plan you create with your dietitian should also take into account your lifestyle, food preferences, and culture. If you're a vegetarian or if you can't eat certain foods for religious reasons, for example, your meal plan needs to reflect that. If you'll be cooking most of your meals for your family or you work late and don't usually have time to cook, your dietitian can help you find foods and recipes to meet your needs. Because so many different elements go into creating a meal plan, the input of an RD or RDN is helpful.

TIP

When working with your dietitian, take advantage of the wonderful resource at your disposal and ask questions. In addition to helping you develop an individualized meal plan, your dietitian can teach you the basics of diabetes nutrition, give you tips on shopping and eating out, and even help you make some of your favorite recipes healthier. Embrace the process and take the opportunity to learn more about your body and diabetes.

REMEMBER

Ultimately, an effective meal plan is all about balance. It should balance the foods you eat with any diabetes medications you take (including insulin) and your physical activity level to keep your blood glucose levels within a normal range. At the same time, it should help you meet your diabetes goals and still allow you to enjoy your food. A dietitian can help you achieve this kind of balance.

More Than One Way to Plan a Meal

When you work with an RD or RDN, he or she may suggest a few different meal-planning methods for you to consider. No one meal-planning approach works for all people with diabetes. Everyone is different, and there are several meal-planning strategies to explore. Understanding the different options can help you decide, with the help of your dietitian, which of these options suits your needs. Here are the most common meal-planning methods:

>> **Portion control:** This meal-planning method focuses on weighing and measuring foods and estimating portion sizes to ensure that you're eating the correct amount of food. It may be used in conjunction with other meal-planning methods.

>> **The plate method:** This easy meal-planning technique uses a plate divided into sections to teach you the correct types and amounts of foods to enjoy at each meal. It promotes portion control and well-balanced meals. Find out more about this method in Chapter 17.

>> **Carbohydrate counting:** In simplest terms, this meal-planning method refers to tracking the amount of carbohydrate you eat. There is a basic and an advanced version of carbohydrate counting. The version you use will depend on your needs and diabetes goals. Generally speaking, people with diabetes who use insulin practice advanced carbohydrate counting. Chapter 18 gives you more details about carbohydrate counting.

>> **Diabetes food choices/exchanges:** This meal planning system shows the number of food "choices" that people with diabetes should eat at each meal and snack based on the American Diabetes Association and Academy of Nutrition and Dietetics' publication *Choose Your Foods: Food Lists for Diabetes.* The food lists in this guide group together foods that have the about the same amount of carbohydrate, protein, fat, and calories. This approach to meal planning makes choosing between food options and navigating serving sizes even easier. Check out Chapter 19 for more about basing your meal plan on food choices/exchanges.

>> **Diabetes-friendly eating patterns:** Even though there is no specific "diabetes diet" that works for everyone with diabetes, several healthy-eating patterns work well for people with type 2 diabetes. These eating patterns include the Mediterranean-style eating plan, the Dietary Approaches to Stop Hypertension (DASH) eating plan, plant-based (vegetarian/vegan) eating patterns, and low-carbohydrate and low-fat eating patterns. These healthy eating patterns focus more on high-quality, nutrient-dense foods than they do on specific nutrients. Chapter 20 goes into more details about these eating patterns.

REMEMBER

There is no one perfect meal plan for people with diabetes, and the American Diabetes Association does not recommend a specific distribution of carbohydrate, protein, and fat for everyone with diabetes. An effective meal plan should be tailored to fit your needs and goals. So if you don't already have a meal plan, familiarize yourself with the planning methods and eating patterns discussed in Chapters 17–20, and then meet with your dietitian to determine which approach is the best fit for *you.*

Chapter **17**

The Plate Method

I t may seem simple, but portion control is one of the most important aspects of healthy eating with diabetes. Today, portion sizes for packaged and restaurant foods are larger than ever, and many people eat much larger portions than they need without even realizing it. So if losing or maintaining weight is one of your goals, portion control can make a big difference in your diet. Eating the right portion sizes and balanced meals can help with weight and carbohydrate management. Fortunately, a few easy methods can help you put portion control into practice.

The Plate Method, also known as Create Your Plate, is a meal planning strategy that helps to manage portion sizes and promote healthy food choices. In this chapter, we walk you through the steps of the Plate Method and touch on a few other portion control tips. After you understand the basics of the Plate Method, you can ask your healthcare provider or a registered dietitian (RD) or registered dietitian nutritionist (RDN) if this is the right meal-planning strategy for you!

Using the Plate Method

The Plate Method, also known as Create Your Plate, is a straightforward and effective strategy for managing diabetes and losing weight. Unlike some other diabetes meal-planning methods, the Plate Method doesn't require a lot of food label reading or counting; all you need is a dinner plate. This means you can practice the Plate Method just about anywhere you go — at home, in restaurants, even at dinner parties.

There are so many healthy foods for people with diabetes to enjoy, and the Plate Method is a great tool to help you combine these foods in the right proportions to create balanced, nutritious meals. (For more information on healthy food choices, see Chapter 1.)

This method appeals to many people with diabetes because it allows you to eat the foods you choose, but it focuses on the portion sizes with an emphasis on eating more nonstarchy vegetables and less starchy foods and proteins.

In the following sections, we explain the Plate Method and address some common concerns people often have. Then we give you some examples of nonstarchy vegetables, starches, and protein options that will help you build healthy and tasty meals.

Divide and fill

The Plate Method is simple: Take a dinner plate and divide it into sections (either mentally or physically); then fill each section with the appropriate type of food. Want to try it yourself? Using Figure 17–1, follow these easy steps to get started:

1. **Using a dinner plate (approximately 9 inches in diameter), draw an imaginary line down the middle of the plate dividing it in half; then on one side, divide that section in half as well, so you have three sections on your plate.**

2. **Fill the largest section (half of your plate) with nonstarchy vegetables.**

3. **In one of the smaller sections, you can include grains and starchy foods such as brown rice, corn, potatoes, or whole-wheat pasta or bread. Remember that fruit, milk, and yogurt also contain carbohydrate and should be taken into consideration in this section of the plate.**

4. **Fill the other smaller section with your protein.**

5. **Choose healthy fats in small amounts when preparing or serving your meal.**

    For example, use plant-based oils for cooking. Try topping salads with nuts, seeds, avocado, and/or vinaigrettes.

6. **Add a low-calorie or zero-calorie drink like water, unsweetened tea, or black coffee to your meal.**

It's that simple! By filling most of your plate with nonstarchy vegetables and eating smaller portions of starches and proteins, you can reduce your calorie, fat, and carbohydrate intake and enjoy more balanced meals.

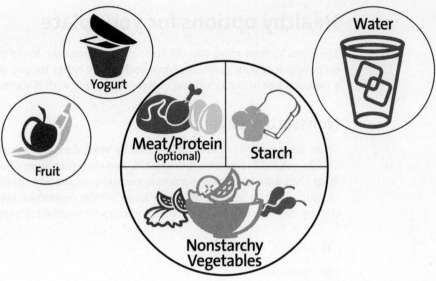

Courtesy of the American Diabetes Association

FIGURE 17-1:
The Plate Method is an easy way to manage diabetes and lose or maintain your weight.

What about breakfast?

Most people don't eat a lot of nonstarchy vegetables for breakfast, so you may be wondering how you use the Plate Method at breakfast time. You may not need to follow the Plate Method exactly at breakfast. But even if you're not enjoying vegetables as part of your meal, the Plate Method can still be helpful. Keeping the Plate Method in mind during breakfast can help you choose appropriate portions of leans proteins and starchy foods.

Choose healthy options from at least a few different food groups when deciding what to eat for breakfast. Breakfast is an important part of your day and can help keep your appetite in check the rest of the day. And don't forget — plenty of recipes incorporate nonstarchy vegetables into breakfast dishes! Try a delicious egg white omelet with spinach, or a fruit-and-vegetable smoothie.

Where do combination foods fit?

Many foods, like lasagna, chili, and stews, are made up of some combination of proteins, starches, and vegetables. So where do these foods fit into the Plate Method? A good rule of thumb is to put combination foods on half of your plate, and make sure you fill the rest of the plate with nonstarchy vegetables. Or, depending on the dish, you can incorporate a large portion of nonstarchy vegetables into the combination food. If you're making bean, meat, and veggie chili, for example, make sure you add those ingredients in proportions similar to the Plate Method — about half of the chili should be nonstarchy vegetables.

Healthy options for your plate

The Plate Method gives you the freedom to choose the foods you want to add to each section of your plate. But some options are better for you than others. Here's a look at a few of the healthiest choices for people with diabetes.

Nonstarchy vegetables

There are two types of vegetables: starchy vegetables and nonstarchy vegetables. Starchy vegetables contain more starch, and therefore more calories and carbohydrate than nonstarchy vegetables. Nonstarchy vegetables should fill the majority of your plate, so it's important to know which vegetables are considered nonstarchy. Some examples of common nonstarchy vegetables include

>> Arugula

>> Asparagus

>> Brussels sprouts

>> Broccoli

>> Cabbage

>> Carrots

>> Cauliflower

>> Celery

>> Cucumber

>> Endive

>> Escarole

>> Green beans

>> Lettuce

>> Mushrooms

>> Onions

>> Peppers

>> Radicchio

>> Romaine

>> Spinach

>> Squash

- » Tomatoes

- » Watercress

- » Zucchini

These are just a few of the nonstarchy vegetables you can enjoy! So fill half of your plate with a refreshing and colorful salad, some sautéed green beans or mushrooms, some roasted Brussels sprouts — or whatever nonstarchy vegetables you love.

REMEMBER

A few vegetables are considered starchy foods, and they should make up only a small section of your plate if you're using the Plate Method. Some examples of starchy vegetables include potatoes, corn, peas, and acorn and butternut squash. Starchy vegetable are still an important part of a healthy diet, but they should be eaten in moderation.

Grains and starchy foods

When using the Plate Method, one-quarter of your plate is reserved for starchy foods. Although starches should be enjoyed in moderation, healthy starches can add vitamins and fiber to your diet. Many of us are used to eating refined starches such as white breads, rice, and pastas; these starches add calories and carbohydrate to your meal without adding many vitamins, minerals, or other nutrients. Choosing healthier whole-grain starches, starchy vegetables, or beans and legumes allows you to get more nutrients from the starchy foods section of your plate.

Nutrient-rich starch options include

- » Beans

- » Corn

- » Lentils

- » Peas

- » Potatoes, white and sweet

- » Rice, brown and wild

- » Whole grains, such as barley, bulgur, faro, millet, oats, and quinoa

- » Whole-wheat or whole-grain breads and pastas

Make the most of your starches by selecting one of these options instead of refined grain products.

Protein

There are several healthy protein options for people with diabetes. The goal when choosing protein is to look for lean cuts of meat and poultry, seafood such as fresh fish, or plant-based proteins such as beans and legumes or soy products. Try to avoid products that have been fried or cooked with a lot of fat.

When it comes to poultry, white meat cuts such as breasts and tenderloins with the skin removed are the best options. Seafood is a great lean protein option for people with diabetes; fish that are rich in omega-3 fatty acids — such as albacore tuna, salmon, herring, sardines, and mackerel — are great choices. Many cuts of red meat and pork contain more fat than other types of protein. Look for lean cuts of meat that have been trimmed of excess fat, and try to avoid high-fat, highly processed meats like bacon, sausage, ground beef, and hot dogs.

Plant-based proteins — for example, beans, lentils, chickpeas, meat substitutes, and tofu and tempeh — are excellent options for people with diabetes. In addition to providing protein, many of these proteins also provide fiber and healthy fats. But keep in mind that plant-based proteins also contain carbohydrate.

More Portion Control Advice

The Plate Method is a simple and effective way to keep portion sizes in check, build healthy meals, and work more nonstarchy vegetables into your diet. But if weight loss is one of your diabetes goals, you may be interested in a few additional portion control tips to help keep you on track.

Simple portion size estimation guidelines

TIP

Identifying the correct portion for some everyday food items is a piece of cake if you use common household items as guidelines. These household items make great visualization tools; if you're familiar with the size of these items, you can estimate how much of the corresponding food to serve yourself and your family. Here are a few of the most common portion size estimation guidelines:

>> 1 teaspoon = about the size of your fingertip

>> 1 tablespoon = about the size of your thumb

>> 3 ounces meat, fish, poultry = the palm of your hand or 1 deck of cards

>> 1 ounce cheese = about the size of your thumb or a pair of dice

>> 1 cup milk, yogurt, or vegetables = the size of a tennis ball

>> 1 medium piece fruit = the size of a tennis ball or an average-size fist

These guidelines will help you visualize correct portion sizes for the foods listed. For other foods and beverages, it's a good idea to use measuring cups and spoons for a while to acclimate yourself to the right serving sizes. For example, measure out one serving of your favorite healthy breakfast cereal, and pour it into a bowl. Pay attention to how that amount of cereal looks in your bowl. A food scale may also be helpful. Eventually you'll be able to eyeball the correct serving without measuring.

It's easy to train your brain to recognize correct portion sizes; after a week or two you probably won't need to use measuring tools or household items to estimate serving sizes. Most people find that, over time, their portions start creeping back up to where they were before they began practicing portion control. When this happens, it's a good idea to go back to weighing or measuring your foods for a few days to get back on track.

TIP

Some people find it helpful to track the portions they eat for a few days before starting to use any portion control techniques. Simply keep a record of the all food you eat for about 3 days, using a food tracker or pen and paper. Then you can compare the amount of food you normally eat to the actual serving sizes on packages or to the portion size guidelines listed earlier. You may find that you've been eating more than you thought.

Portion control tips

Even with the Plate Method and portion size estimation techniques in your arsenal, you may still be tempted to overeat in certain situations. Here are a few tips to make it easier to avoid temptation:

>> Instead of serving family meals at the table, serve the food in the kitchen and bring it out to the table. If the leftover food is out of sight, you may be less tempted to reach for a second serving.

>> Your body may not recognize that it's full right away. Eat slowly and savor your food as you're eating. Take a break between bites and give yourself time to realize that you're full.

>> It's easy to overeat at parties; food is often all around and it's easy to grab a little at a time without realizing how much you're eating. If you eat a light, healthy snack before heading to a party, you may be less likely to overeat.

» It's especially difficult to control portion sizes when snacking. Many people end up eating several servings of their snack of choice without realizing it. To prevent this, measure out one serving of snack foods instead of eating directly out of the package. Try to avoid eating mindlessly in front of the TV or computer — pay attention to your body so you know when you're full.

» If you have specific foods you tend to overeat, don't buy those foods anymore, or at least store them somewhere out of sight. Out of sight, out of mind.

With a little planning and a few simple tips, tricks, and strategies, you'll be a master of portion control in no time!

Chapter **18**

Carbohydrate Counting

I f you've been diagnosed with diabetes or prediabetes, you've probably heard a *lot* of talk about carbohydrate. Carbohydrate is an important nutrient for people with diabetes to understand because it's the nutrient that has the most impact on your blood glucose levels after meals. When you eat carbohydrate-containing foods, your body breaks carbohydrate down into several different types of simple sugars including glucose, which your body uses for energy. The glucose enters your bloodstream, and your blood glucose levels start to rise. Your body needs some glucose in order to function properly; however, if people with diabetes eat too much carbohydrate, their blood glucose can rise well above normal levels. Over time, high blood glucose can cause dangerous side effects. So it's essential that people with diabetes manage their carbohydrate intake. In fact, carbohydrate control is one of the most important aspects of any diabetes meal plan.

In this chapter, we explore the diabetes meal planning method that deals directly with managing carbohydrate intake: carbohydrate counting. Carbohydrate counting simply means tracking the amount of carbohydrate you eat. To get started with carbohydrate counting, you need to know which foods contain carbohydrate and how much carbohydrate your body needs each day. Then we walk you through the carbohydrate counting basics and even touch on some advanced carbohydrate counting techniques.

REMEMBER

Eating foods that contain carbohydrate will cause your blood glucose to rise, but carbohydrate is the main source of fuel for your body and can provide some essential vitamins, minerals, and fiber (if you choose nutritious carbohydrate foods). You don't need to completely eliminate carbohydrate from your diet. Instead focus on choosing healthy sources of carbohydrate and managing your intake of carbohydrate-rich foods.

Know Your Carbs

Because carbohydrate has such a big impact on your blood glucose levels, it's important to understand the sources of carbohydrate in our diets. Where does carbohydrate come from? It may surprise you to learn that carbohydrate is found in a wide variety of foods — some very nutritious, others a bit less healthy. Foods that contain carbohydrate or "carbs" include

>> Fruit

>> Fruit juices

>> Starchy vegetables, such as corn, peas, potatoes, and pumpkin

>> Beans

>> Lentils

>> Soy-based foods, such as meat substitutes, tempeh, tofu, and veggie burgers

>> Milk

>> Yogurt

>> Grains, such as oatmeal, quinoa, barley, farro, and rice

>> Grain-based foods, such as bread, cereals, pasta, and crackers

>> Sweets and snack foods, such as cake, candy, cookies, chips, and regular sodas

Nonstarchy vegetables — such as tomatoes, carrots, peppers, broccoli, and salad greens — also contain carbohydrate. However, they are very low in carbohydrate and can be enjoyed in relatively large quantities with minimal impact on blood glucose. So, don't be afraid to add some tasty nonstarchy veggies to your plate!

TIP

When choosing carbohydrate foods, look for nutrient-rich options like fruits, vegetables, beans and legumes, and whole-grains. These options contain fiber and other important nutrients that processed and refined sources of carbohydrate may not provide. Try to limit your intake of processed carbohydrates such as white breads, white pasta, sugary desserts, and regular sodas.

How Much Carbohydrate Is Right For Me?

The first step to carbohydrate counting is to figure out how many grams of carbohydrate your body needs each day and at each meal. Once you have carbohydrate goals in place, you can begin tracking the amount of carbohydrate you eat to make sure you don't exceed your goals.

In order to better understand and work toward your carbohydrate goals, it can be helpful to first honestly track the amount of carbohydrate in what you normally eat throughout the day. Many people may find that they're already within their carbohydrate goals at some meals, but there may be one meal or time of day where what they normally eat exceeds their carbohydrate goals. When they know this, they can focus on meeting their carbohydrate goals for that meal first; this is a good starting point that can provide a lot of benefit in terms of blood glucose management without feeling too overwhelming.

The American Diabetes Association doesn't recommend a certain amount or range of carbohydrate that all people with diabetes should aim for each day. The amount of carbohydrate that is right for you is based on your individual needs. Determining the right amount for you depends on many different factors including your physical activity level; your eating patterns; your culture, lifestyle, and preferences; and what, if any, medicines you take. The amount of carbohydrate you eat per day should also help you achieve your diabetes goals; for example, if you want to lose weight in addition to lowering your blood glucose, your carbohydrate goals should take that into account. Some people can eat more carbohydrate than others and still keep their blood glucose levels in their target range. Finding the right balance of carbohydrate for you can provide you more control over blood glucose levels, potentially lower your risk of diabetes complications, and help you feel your best.

TIP

Discuss your personal carbohydrate needs with a registered dietitian (RD) or registered dietitian nutritionist (RDN) or your diabetes care team. A diabetes nutrition professional can help you determine how many grams of carbohydrate are right for you per day, how to split those grams between your meals, and if and where snacks might fit in your daily carbohydrate goals.

REMEMBER

Your carbohydrate needs may change over time. You may need to adjust your carbohydrate goals if your weight, activity level, or medications change. As your diabetes progresses, it may become more difficult to manage your blood glucose using the same methods you first did and your carbohydrate goals may need to change at certain meals or over the course of the day. Don't be afraid to reevaluate your carbohydrate intake with your healthcare team!

Basic Carbohydrate Counting: Be Consistent

Carbohydrate counting is really just a way to keep track of the amount of carbohydrate you're eating. But there are actually two methods of carbohydrate counting: basic and advanced.

The goal of basic carbohydrate counting is consistency. People who follow a basic carbohydrate counting plan will have a target number of carbohydrate grams to aim for at each meal and snack. If you're using this method of carbohydrate counting, eating around the same times each day and knowing how many carbs to eat at each of those times is the goal. Your carbohydrate goals may be different for breakfast, lunch, and dinner, but you have a goal for each meal and try to stay within that range.

REMEMBER

Although the amount and timing of your carbohydrate intake should stay consistent with basic carbohydrate counting, you're encouraged to eat a variety of healthy foods.

You can enjoy any carbohydrate-containing food as long as you account for it in your meal plan. If you practice basic carbohydrate counting, you'll read the label on the food to determine how many grams of carbohydrate are in a serving and how many servings you actually want to eat of that food to get to your goal. You can keep a record of the amount of carbohydrate you eat at each meal using any method that works best for you. Some people like using a diabetes logbook, others like simple pen and paper, and others prefer using a food-tracking program or mobile applications. It's a good idea to keep a record of what you eat, especially the amount of carbohydrate you eat, for a few days or a week prior to an appointment with your doctor or dietitian. That way if there are any changes in your blood glucose levels, you'll have a record of your eating patterns.

TIP

It's important to pay attention to serving sizes when you're counting carbohydrate. If you double the serving size of a food, you double the amount of carbohydrate you're eating. Eating more carbohydrate than you normally do at a meal will likely make your blood glucose level higher than usual after several hours. It's a good idea to measure your foods with measuring cups and spoons if you're not sure exactly what 1 cup of soup or ⅔ cup of yogurt looks like.

This basic counting strategy works for many people with diabetes, especially those with type 2 diabetes. Why? Because if you eat about the same amount of carbohydrate at each meal and snack, your blood glucose levels should become a bit more predictable. Reducing fluctuations in blood glucose levels can help lower your risk for diabetes complications and keep you feeling strong and healthy.

Basic carbohydrate counting can also help you notice trends in how your body reacts to carbohydrate foods. *Note:* Other factors besides the carbohydrate you eat can affect your blood glucose; keep that in mind if your blood glucose readings are not what you expected.

TIP

The basic carbohydrate counting method is a meal-planning approach that generally works for people who can manage their blood glucose with diet and exercise alone or take fixed doses of insulin. Ask your healthcare provider if this meal-planning method is right for you.

Advanced Carbohydrate Counting

Advanced carbohydrate counting is more precise than the basic method. With advanced carbohydrate counting, you track the exact number of carbohydrate grams in the foods you eat. This method of carbohydrate counting is often used by people who are on insulin — usually multiple daily injections or an insulin pump — and need to match the amount of carbohydrate they consume to an insulin dose. Knowing the exact amount of carbohydrate you eat at each meal makes calculating insulin injections easier and more accurate. Discuss your needs with your healthcare team to determine if this method of carbohydrate counting is right for you.

REMEMBER

As with basic carbohydrate counting (see the preceding section), the advanced method of carbohydrate counting allows you more freedom to choose which carbohydrate-containing foods you'd like to eat. But in both cases it's important to still follow basic nutrition principles and balance your carbohydrate intake with healthy proteins, fats, and nonstarchy vegetables. You also want to be calorie conscious when you practice carbohydrate counting if you're trying to lose or maintain your weight. Don't let the focus on carbohydrate distract you from good nutrition!

Calculating specific carbohydrate amounts

Advance carbohydrate counting is a little more complex than the basic method and requires some basic math skills, especially for people who are using insulin. People who practice advanced carbohydrate counting use food labels to calculate the amount of carbohydrate in the foods they're eating. It's a good idea to familiarize yourself with the Nutrition Facts panel on food labels (see Figure 18-1). The nutrition information in this panel is the most accurate tool to use when calculating the amount of carbohydrate in your foods.

Nutrition Facts

8 servings per container

Serving size   **2/3 cup (55g)**

Amount per serving

Calories   230

% Daily Value*

Total Fat 8g	**10%**
Saturated Fat 1g	**5%**
Trans Fat 0g	
Cholesterol 0mg	**0%**
Sodium 160mg	**7%**
Total Carbohydrate 37g	**13%**
Dietary Fiber 4g	**14%**
Total Sugars 12g	
Includes 10g Added Sugars	**20%**
Protein 3g	
Vitamin D 2mcg	10%
Calcium 260mcg	20%
Iron 8mg	45%
Potassium 235mg	6%

*The % Daily Value (DV) tells you how much a nutrient in a serving of food contributes to a daily diet. 2,000 calories a day is used for general nutrition advice.

FIGURE 18-1:
A standard
Nutrition Facts
panel.

Courtesy of the American Diabetes Association

When you've determined the grams of carbohydrate in your meal, write the number down! Keeping track of the total grams of carbohydrate that you eat at each meal or snack is very important if you practice advanced carbohydrate counting. These values can help you calculate insulin doses, if you use insulin, and may help you troubleshoot inconsistencies in your blood glucose. So keep a written or electronic record for your own uses and to share with your healthcare provider.

TIP

If you use multiple daily injections of insulin or an insulin pump and you're having trouble matching your insulin doses to your carbohydrate intake, it's important to make an appointment with a diabetes educator or a doctor. These professionals can help you calculate how many units of insulin you'll need to balance out the carbohydrate you eat.

Now that you know the basics of advanced carbohydrate counting, let's take a look at a few methods to figure out the amount of carbohydrate in your foods: using nutrition labels and performing some advanced calculations.

Using nutrition panels

When you're reading food labels for carbohydrate-counting purposes, the two most important lines in the Nutrition Facts panel are the serving size and the total carbohydrate. To determine the amount of carbohydrate in the food you're eating, follow these simple steps:

1. **Locate the serving size on the nutrition panel.**

All of the nutrition information on the nutrition panel is based on this serving of the food. If you eat more or less of the food than the serving size listed, the amount of each nutrient you're consuming will be different than listed. For example, if you eat two servings of the food, you will need to double the information on the label.

2. **Locate the amount of "Total Carbohydrate."**

The grams of total carbohydrate given are for the serving size listed. The amount of total carbohydrate on the nutrition panel includes the sugar, starch, and fiber in that food.

3. **Know your carbohydrate goal for your meal, and adjust how much you eat of the food to meet your goal.**

For example, say you eat 15 grams of carbohydrate for a snack each afternoon. You would like to eat 1 cup of pretzels as your snack, but you read the nutrition label and see that total carbohydrate grams for ½ cup of pretzels is 30 grams. You can serve yourself a half serving of pretzels (¼ cup) so you don't exceed your carbohydrate goal. If you eat ½ cup of pretzels, your blood glucose will likely be higher afterward than if you eat the ¼-cup portion that meets your carbohydrate goal.

Reading nutrition labels can be confusing at first, but it gets easier with practice. There are a few common mistakes that people make when learning to calculate carbohydrate grams using food labels that you should be aware of:

>> People often confuse the grams of sugar on the nutrition label for the grams of total carbohydrate, so they only count the sugar grams of their meal and often end up underestimating their carbohydrate intake.

>> Some people may mistake the total grams of food they're eating (listed after the serving size) for the grams of carbohydrate.

>> Some people add the number of sugar grams listed on the label to the total carbohydrate grams and end up overestimating their carbohydrate intake.

These common missteps can be avoided by remembering that the total carbohydrate value on the nutrition label already includes the sugar, fiber, and starch in that food. By counting the total carbohydrate grams, you're taking into account all of the ingredients that have the most impact on blood glucose. So, generally speaking, the total carbohydrate grams and serving size will be your focus when counting carbohydrate.

REMEMBER

You won't find a Nutrition Facts panel on every food you eat. For foods that don't have labels — such as fresh produce or restaurant foods — there are many online food databases available to help you find out how much carbohydrate is in a serving of the food. The U.S. Department of Agriculture, for example, has an online tool called SuperTracker (http://supertracker.usda.gov) that can help you find the nutrients in foods without labels. Many diabetes-friendly cookbooks, including all cookbooks published by the American Diabetes Association, provide nutrition information for recipes so you don't have to estimate the nutrient content of these dishes on your own. As a quick reference, we've included carbohydrate grams for a few common foods:

>> ½ cup of blueberries = 11 grams

>> 1 small orange = 11 grams

>> 1 small apple = 15 grams

>> ½ cup grapes = 15 grams

>> 1 small banana = 23 grams

>> ½ cup of cooked green peas = 11 grams

>> 1 medium ear of corn = 20 grams

>> ½ baked acorn squash = 14 grams

>> 1 plain baked potato or sweet potato = about 35–40 grams

>> ½ cup cooked macaroni noodles = 21 grams

>> ½ cup cooked brown rice = 22 grams

>> ½ cup mashed potatoes = 23 grams

TIP

You may be interested in a few other features of the nutrition panel as well, depending on your other health and diabetes management goals:

>> **Calories:** Keep an eye on the amount of calories you're eating, especially if you're trying to lose or maintain weight.

>> **Saturated and trans fats:** Minimize the amount of saturated fat you eat and look for foods with 0 grams of trans fat. This is especially important for people who have an increased risk for cardiovascular complications such as heart disease and stroke.

>> **Sodium:** People who are concerned about their blood pressure may benefit from reducing the amount of sodium they eat. Compare information on nutrition labels and look for products with the lowest amount of sodium.

REMEMBER

Remember that the information given on the nutrition label is based on the serving size listed; if you eat a portion that is more or less than the serving size, you'll need to adjust the nutrition information accordingly.

Getting (even more) technical

For people who practice advanced carbohydrate counting, tracking the total carbohydrate grams in their foods is key; these numbers allow them to manage their blood glucose levels and calculate insulin doses (if needed). The "Total Carbohydrate" value on nutrition panels accounts for all types of carbohydrate in the food — including sugars, dietary fiber, and sugar alcohols — but not all types of carbohydrate affect your blood glucose in the exact same way. Dietary fiber and sugar alcohols may have less of an impact on blood glucose than other forms of carbohydrate, such as sugars and starches. Let's explore how these two types of carbohydrate affect your body and your meal plan.

Dietary fiber is a part of plant foods that either isn't digested or is only partially digested by the body when eaten. Fiber is found in fruits, vegetables, grains, beans, and legumes. Fiber helps maintain digestive health and may help you feel full and satisfied after eating. Women should aim to eat 25 grams of fiber per day, and men should aim for 38 grams per day. Many people only get about half of the fiber they need per day. Because fiber isn't fully digested, you may want to talk to your dietitian or diabetes care team about how fiber may impact your insulin needs, especially if you're eating a lot of fiber.

Sugar alcohols are reduced-calorie sweeteners used in many foods including "sugar-free" food. Some common sugar alcohols include erythritol, isomalt, xylitol, mannitol, sorbitol, lactitol, and hydrogenated starch hydrolysates. Sugar alcohols contain one-half of the calories of other sweeteners and may cause smaller increases in blood glucose after eating than other types of carbohydrate, but they still have an impact.

Sugar alcohols are safe to eat in moderate amounts. But products that contain sugar alcohols, when eaten in excess, may cause gastrointestinal symptoms such as cramping and diarrhea. It's also important to note that just because a food contains sugar alcohols or is labeled "sugar-free" doesn't mean it's free of carbohydrate. Use caution when selecting and eating these foods.

REMEMBER

When it comes to carbohydrate counting, it's the total carbohydrate grams (not the grams of sugar, fiber, or sugar alcohols) that are important. Consult with your dietitian or diabetes care team to see if and how fiber and sugar alcohols affect your insulin needs.

Chapter **19**

Meal Planning with Food Choices/Exchanges

One of the most important things to remember when you're trying to adopt a diabetes-friendly diet is that there is no one-size-fits-all meal plan that works for all people with diabetes. The meal planning method you use should be selected with the help of a registered dietitian (RD) or registered dietitian nutritionist (RDN) based on your preferences, lifestyle, and diabetes and other health goals. Some people enjoy the ease and simplicity of the Plate Method, while many others find that carbohydrate counting helps them manage their blood glucose levels. (Learn more about the Plate Method and carbohydrate counting in Chapters 17 and 18, respectively.) If you're looking for a little more precision than the Plate Method offers but you don't want to count grams of carbohydrate, meal planning with food choices may be the right method for you.

Food choices (sometimes called exchanges) can be a helpful meal-planning tool for some people with diabetes. This meal-planning approach is based on the American Diabetes Association and Academy of Nutrition and Dietetics' booklet *Choose Your Foods: Food Lists for Diabetes,* a collection of categorized food lists. These food lists, formerly called exchange lists, group foods with a similar nutrient makeup together. Food lists take the guesswork out of choosing the right foods in the correct serving sizes for your meal plan.

This chapter gives you a closer look at the different food lists used in this meal-planning method and explains how you can get started using food choices.

What Are Food Choices?

The term *choice* is used to describe a certain quantity of food within each food list (group of nutritionally similar foods). Each item you see on a food list equals one choice, though the serving size will vary for each food item.

For example, in the Starch food list, one Starch choice is equal to (approximately) ½ cup of cooked grains or starchy vegetables, ⅓ cup of cooked pasta or rice, or 1 ounce of a bread product. If you're using food choices to plan your meals, you can simply choose foods from the food lists that correspond with the amount of choices in your meal plan. So, if your meal plan allows you to have two Starch choices at dinner each night, you can enjoy any two foods or servings of food from the Starch list as part of that meal.

REMEMBER

Pay attention to the serving sizes given in the food lists; those serving sizes represent one choice of that specific type of food. If you increase the serving size, you increase the number of choices you're eating. For example, if ½ cup of cereal equals one Starch choice, then 1 cup of cereal will equal two Starch choices.

REMEMBER

Any food from a certain food list can be replaced with any other food on that same list because all the foods that are grouped together have a similar amount of calories, carbohydrate, fat, and protein. So if you substitute one food item on the Starch list for another, for instance, you'll still be consuming roughly the same amount of carbohydrate.

Getting to Know the Food Lists

There are several categories of food lists — including proteins; fats; fruits, non-starchy vegetables, and other carbohydrates; combination foods; and even fast foods — to help you create balanced meals in any situation. In the following sections, we look at the food options included in these different categories and the nutrient profiles of each list. This should give you an idea of whether meal planning with food choices/exchanges is the right approach for you. The complete set of food lists is available in the appendix.

Starch

The Starch food list covers a variety of different starchy foods. This is the list where you'll find foods that will have the greatest impact on your blood glucose. Whole grains (such as brown rice, oats, and quinoa), pastas, cereals, bread products, many desserts, and crackers, pretzels, and other starchy snacks can all be found on the Starch list. Starchy vegetables, such as potatoes, corn, green peas, beans, acorn squash, and pumpkin, are included in this list because they are higher in carbohydrate than nonstarchy vegetables.

REMEMBER

When choosing foods from the Starch list, remember that starchy vegetables, whole grains, and beans (which contain vitamins, minerals, and fiber) are more nutritious choices than processed, refined starches such as white breads and pastas, and sugary desserts.

REMEMBER

Starchy foods that are prepared with fat, such as baked goods or starchy vegetables, count as one Starch choice and one Fat choice.

One Starch choice contains 15 grams of carbohydrate, 3 grams of protein, 1 gram of fat, and 80 calories. Generally speaking, one Starch choice is equal to

>> ½ cup of cooked grains or starchy vegetables

>> ⅓ cup of cooked rice or pasta

>> 1 ounce of bread (bread products that are larger than 1 ounce will equal more than one choice)

>> ¾–1 ounce of starchy snack foods

Fruits

The Fruits list covers all types and preparations of fruit, including fresh, frozen, dried, and canned fruits and fruit juices. When you purchase canned fruits, you'll notice that there are several types of canning liquids used: juice, light, syrup, and heavy syrup. All the canned fruits on the Fruits list are either "no sugar added," "juice pack," or canned in extra-light syrup. All three of these options have a similar amount of carbohydrate, and they're the best canned fruit options for people with diabetes. Fruits canned in heavy syrup should be avoided.

One Fruit choice contains 15 grams of carbohydrate, 0 grams of protein and fat, and 60 calories. In terms of portion sizes, one Fruit choice is the equivalent of

>> ½ cup of canned or frozen fruit

>> 1 small piece of fresh fruit

>> ½ cup of fruit juice (unsweetened)

>> 2 tablespoons of dried fruit

Some of the whole fresh fruits on the Fruits list are measured by weight (rind and seeds included) instead of cups or tablespoons. It's a good idea to weigh your fresh fruits using a food scale to get an idea of the size of your favorite fruits and how that relates to the number of choices you'll be eating. Fruits are full of beneficial nutrients, but they also contain carbohydrate, so serving size matters!

Milk and Milk Substitutes

The Milk and Milk Substitutes list includes a variety of different milk options, including rice and soy milks and yogurt. But not all dairy products are included on this list; you'll find items like cheese, butter, cream, nut milks, and ice cream on other food lists because they contain minimal carbohydrate and, therefore, don't impact your blood glucose like milk and milk substitutes will.

The best Milk and Milk Substitute choices for people with diabetes are usually lower-fat varieties such as fat-free or low-fat milk, or low-fat or nonfat yogurt.

One Milk/Milk Substitute choice contains 12 grams of carbohydrate and 8 grams of protein. The fat and calorie content varies among the items on this list. For example:

>> Fat-free or low-fat choices contain 0–3 grams of fat and about 100 calories per serving

>> Reduced-fat or 2 percent choices contain 5 grams of fat and 120 calories per serving

>> High-fat or whole-milk choices contain 8 grams of fat and 160 calories per serving

Pay close attention to the fat content and serving size of the foods you choose from this list so you don't consume more carbohydrate, fat, and calories than you intend to.

Nonstarchy Vegetables

This food list is made up of raw, canned, and cooked nonstarchy vegetables including tomatoes, onions, mushrooms, broccoli, carrots, spinach, summer squash, and zucchini (to name just a few). Because they're higher in carbohydrate and calories, starchy vegetables such as corn, green peas, potatoes, and winter squash are included in the Starch list.

TIP

Nonstarchy vegetables are an important part of a diabetes-friendly meal plan, and you should aim to eat several servings of these vegetables each day. If you choose canned vegetables or vegetable juice, look for no-salt-added or low-sodium options. If you can't find low-sodium canned vegetables, drain and rinse them before use to reduce their sodium content.

One Nonstarchy Vegetable choice contains 5 grams of carbohydrate, 2 grams of protein, 0 grams of fat, and 25 calories. In general, one Nonstarchy Vegetable choice equals

>> ½ cup of cooked vegetables

>> 1 cup of raw vegetables

>> ½ cup of vegetable juice

TECHNICAL STUFF

Nonstarchy vegetables are low in carbohydrate and can be enjoyed in relatively large quantities. However, if you decide to eat three Nonstarchy Vegetables choices (3 cups of raw vegetables or 1½ cups cooked vegetables or more) in a single meal, you should count them as one Carbohydrate choice instead.

Sweets, Desserts, and Other Carbohydrates

The Sweets, Desserts, and Other Carbohydrates list includes carbohydrate-rich foods that do not have the same nutrient makeup as the foods in the Starch list. This list contains a wide variety of food items including sodas, sports drinks, and other beverages; cakes and cookies; candies and sweeteners; condiments; pastries; and frozen desserts. People with diabetes should select foods from this list less often than other carbohydrate-containing foods such as starches, fruits, and nonstarchy vegetables — all of which contain more fiber and beneficial nutrients than foods on the Sweets, Desserts, and Other Carbohydrates list.

One choice from the Sweets, Desserts, and Other Carbohydrates list (called a Carbohydrate choice) contains 15 grams of carbohydrate and 70 calories. In terms of their carbohydrate, fat, and calorie content, the foods on this list vary widely. In fact, many of the foods on this list contain more than a single Carbohydrate choice, and some include Fat choices as well (one Fat choice is equal to 5 grams of fat and 45 calories).

The Sweets, Desserts, and Other Carbohydrates list specifies how many choices each food contains per serving, so don't worry! You won't have to figure this out on your own.

Protein

The Protein list covers all kinds of protein foods, not just meats, poultry, and fish. Eggs, cheese, and plant-based proteins are also included in the list due to their high protein content. Foods on the Protein list are divided into four groups based on their fat content: lean protein, medium-fat protein, high-fat protein, and plant-based protein. The nutrients in a Protein choice vary based on the type of protein. For example:

>> One lean Protein choice contains 0 grams of carbohydrate, 7 grams of protein, 2 grams of fat, and 45 calories.

>> One medium-fat Protein choice contains 0 grams of carbohydrate, 7 grams of protein, 5 gram of fat, and 75 calories.

>> One high-fat Protein choice contains 0 grams of carbohydrate, 7 grams of protein, 8 grams of fat, and 100 calories.

>> One plant-based Protein choice contains 7 grams of protein just like the other Protein choices, but the amounts of carbohydrate, fat, and calories vary depending on the specific food item. (Note that veggie and soy burgers and other meat substitutes may contain a significant amount of carbohydrate.)

TIP

The best animal Protein choices for people with diabetes are lean meats. Look for lean cuts of meat and poultry when shopping; they contain less saturated fat and cholesterol than higher-fat proteins, such as processed meats and prime cuts.

Don't forget to watch your portion sizes with proteins! The serving sizes given in the Protein list are based on the cooked weight of the protein after bones and excess fat have been removed.

Fats

Like the Protein list, the Fats list is divided into subgroups as well. But in this case, the groups are based on the *type* of fat the foods contain, not the quantity of fat. These three groups are

>> **Unsaturated fats,** which primarily come from plant sources such as nuts and seeds.

>> **Saturated fats,** which primarily come from animal sources and should be consumed in moderation.

>> **Trans fats,** which are a product of food processing; these fats should be avoided.

One Fat choice contains 5 grams of fat and 45 calories, and one choice is equal to approximately

>> 1 teaspoon of oils or solid fats

>> 1 tablespoon of salad dressing

REMEMBER

For the most nutritious fat options, try to choose sources of unsaturated fat from this list over saturated and trans fats whenever you can, and use liquid fats instead of solid fats when cooking.

You may be surprised to see nuts and seeds on the Fats list, but they're a good source of unsaturated fats and contain other beneficial nutrients. Keep in mind, though, that *all fats*, even unsaturated fats, should be eaten in moderation because they're high in calories. So keep an eye on your portion sizes.

Free Foods

A *free food* is defined as any food (or beverage) that contains less than 20 calories and 5 grams of carbohydrate or less per serving. Free foods shouldn't have a significant effect on your blood glucose levels, and you don't need to account for these foods in your meal plan. You'll see a wide variety of foods on this list, from chewing gum and sugar substitutes to reduced-fat mayonnaise and salad dressings to salad greens and small servings of nonstarchy vegetables.

Many of the food items on the Free Foods list have serving sizes, while others don't. Why is that? If a free food is listed with a serving size, it means that the calories and/or carbohydrate in that serving size are close to the limits for a free food. Avoid eating more than three servings of that food per day, and if you choose to eat all three of those servings at once, count them as one Carbohydrate choice. Foods on the Free Foods list without a serving size can be enjoyed at any time.

Combination Foods

Using food choices is simple when you're eating individual foods, but maybe you're wondering where your favorite casserole, soup, or frozen meals fits into this meal-planning method. How do you figure out the choices for foods that are a combination of starches, proteins, fruits or vegetables, and fats? These "combination foods" don't fit clearly into any one food list.

Fortunately, the booklet *Choose Your Foods: Food Lists for Diabetes* provides a Combination Foods list to help with this situation. This list gives the serving size and choices for some typical combination foods that you may encounter, including casseroles, stews and soups, frozen meals, and pizza.

WARNING

If you have favorite combination foods that you prepare at home using your own recipes, the nutrients of those dishes may differ from the information presented in the Combination Foods list. It may be worth doing a little math to figure out the nutrient content of your recipe and find the appropriate exchanges. Your dietitian should be able to help you with this if you bring the recipe to an appointment, or you can work this out on your own following these steps:

1. **Find the amount of calories, carbohydrate, protein, and fat in each ingredient.**

2. **Add up the total amount of calories and the total amount of each other nutrient for the recipe.**

3. **Divide the total amount of calories and the totals for the other nutrients by the number of servings in the dish.**

   This will give you the nutrients for each serving.

4. **Compare the nutrients per serving with the definitions of Carbohydrate, Protein, and Starch choices to determine the choices per serving.**

Fast Foods

Healthy eating doesn't stop when you're on the go! If you're having a busy day and need to stop at a fast-food restaurant for a meal, you can use the Fast Foods list to work that meal into your meal plan. The choices in this list don't represent specific fast food menu items; instead they're estimated based on popular fast-food items. For example, you won't find the choices for a four-piece fried chicken meal from your favorite fast-food restaurant, but you will find entries for breaded and fried chicken breasts, thighs, wings, and drumsticks.

TIP

The Fast Foods list is a great starting point, but if you want the nutrition information for menu items at a specific restaurant, they should be available online.

Making Food Choices/Exchanges Work for You

Now that you're familiar with the food lists in *Choose Your Foods: Food Lists for Diabetes* and you have a better understanding of how food choices/exchanges work, you're ready to put this meal-planning method into practice!

The first and most important step when adopting a meal-planning method is meeting with a dietitian who will help you create an individualized plan. Before you can begin using food choices, you need to know how many choices from each food list is appropriate for you to eat at each meal. That is where an RD or RDN comes in; an RD or RDN can evaluate your lifestyle, eating patterns, blood glucose levels, and diabetes and other health goals and use that information to help you determine how many Starch, Fruit, Nonstarchy Vegetable, Protein, Fat, Milk, and Carbohydrate choices you should eat for each meal and snack (if snacks are part of your plan).

When you know the type and amount of food choices you need to aim for at each meal, you can use the food lists as your guide to select food options that fit into your meal plan. For example, if your goal is to include one Starch choice, two Protein choices, two Nonstarchy Vegetable choices, and one Fat choice in your dinner, you can choose one food from the Starch list, two from the Protein list, two from the Nonstarchy Vegetables list, and one from the Fats list (being sure to add these foods to your plate in the appropriate serving sizes). Make sure you have a copy *Choose Your Foods: Food Lists for Diabetes* available for reference. (See the appendix for the complete collection of food lists.)

Many diabetes-friendly recipes in cookbooks and on the Internet include choices/exchanges for one serving of the recipe to make things convenient for people who practice this method of meal planning. In fact, all the recipes in this book include choices/exchanges as part of the nutrition information. But if you have a favorite recipe that you can't find an equivalent for in the food lists, don't be afraid to ask your dietitian for assistance. He or she should be able to help you determine the calorie and nutrient content of one serving of the food and match those numbers with corresponding food choices. That way you can easily work the food into your meal plan where appropriate.

The ease and flexibility of food choices/exchanges has made this meal-planning method a popular choice among people with diabetes for decades. If you think food choices/exchanges are the right meal-planning tool for you, consult your dietitian.

Chapter **20**

Other Meal Planning Methods

The key to eating well with diabetes is finding a meal plan that meets your personal needs and sets you up to achieve your diabetes goals. There is not one specific "diabetes diet" or meal plan that is right for everyone with diabetes. The Plate Method (see Chapter 17), carbohydrate counting (see Chapter 18), and food choices/exchanges (see Chapter 19) are popular meal planning approaches for people with diabetes, but studies show many different eating patterns can be helpful in managing diabetes. These eating patterns include the Mediterranean-style eating plan, the DASH (Dietary Approaches to Stop Hypertension) eating plan, plant-based (vegetarian/vegan) eating patterns, and low-carbohydrate and low-fat eating patterns. In this chapter, we explore these eating patterns in detail to see if any of them may be right for you.

As you're learning about all the different meal-planning options available, you may come across the terms *glycemic index* and *glycemic load*. We touch briefly on glycemic index and load in this chapter, because they may be useful tools to help you fine-tune your blood glucose management.

Eating Patterns and Meal Planning

An *eating pattern* is the foods or groups of foods that a person chooses to eat on a daily basis over time. According to the American Diabetes Association's *Standards of Medical Care in Diabetes*, a variety of eating patterns are acceptable for the management of type 2 diabetes, including a Mediterranean-style eating pattern, the DASH eating plan, and plant-based eating patterns. These eating patterns place more focus on eating high-quality, nutrient-dense foods than they do on tracking specific nutrients. Low-carbohydrate and low-fat eating patterns may also be appropriate for some people with diabetes. The American Diabetes Association doesn't recommend any one eating plan for people with diabetes; instead, consider these eating patterns as a few of the many healthy eating options for people with diabetes.

REMEMBER

It's important to work with a registered dietitian (RD) or registered dietitian nutritionist (RDN), a physician, or a certified diabetes educator (CDE) to find a meal plan or eating pattern that meets your individual needs. Ultimately, the meal-planning approach that you can follow and sustain in the long run will be the best option for you.

Eating Mediterranean style

The Mediterranean-style eating pattern or diet reflects the way of eating that is typical of people in the areas surrounding the Mediterranean Sea. Studies have shown that people in the Mediterranean region are some of the healthiest in the world. The Mediterranean-style eating pattern focuses mainly on fresh, seasonal, and locally grown plant foods (vegetables, fruits, whole grains, beans, and nuts) and supplements these foods with small amounts of dairy products, fish, and poultry. Fish that are rich in omega-3 fatty acids — such as salmon, albacore tuna, herring, mackerel, and rainbow trout — can be enjoyed a few times per week. Olive oil is the main source of fat used for cooking foods. It's a good source of monounsaturated fat, which can help lower cholesterol when eaten instead of saturated fats (found in butter, margarine, and other solid fats).

People who follow a Mediterranean-style eating pattern are encouraged to limit their consumption of red meat and high-sugar foods. However, wine may be enjoyed in small amounts with a meal if desired. It is recommended that women have no more than one drink per day and men have no more than two drinks per day. One drink or one serving of wine is a 5-ounce glass.

This eating plan's emphasis on plant foods and moderate amounts of dairy, fish, and poultry contrasts with the typical "American diet," which is often full of refined carbohydrates, large portions of proteins (including red meat and processed meats), and lots of fat and sodium. The typical American diet, unlike the Mediterranean-style eating pattern, is lacking in fruits, vegetables, legumes, and whole grains.

The Mediterranean-style eating pattern has been shown to protect against heart disease, stroke, and some types of cancer. Studies have also suggested that this eating pattern may help with weight and blood glucose management, which means it can be considered a good meal-planning option for people with type 2 diabetes. With these potential benefits, it's easy to see why so many people want to follow a Mediterranean lifestyle!

The Mediterranean way of eating is often referred to as the "Mediterranean diet." Many people think of a "diet" as a temporary change in eating habits to bring on some desired result (often weight loss). But the Mediterranean-style eating pattern is more of a way of life than a short-term change to your eating habits. In addition to changing *what* you eat, this eating pattern may change how you think about food and mealtime. If you follow this eating pattern, you'll want to make it a priority to include fresh, seasonal fruits and vegetables in your diet. This may mean planning trips to the farmer's market to ensure you're getting the freshest local ingredients. Another important part of the Mediterranean lifestyle is cooking, eating, and cleaning with family and friends. If you follow this eating pattern, try to make time in your schedule to sit down for a family meal and really enjoy your food and the process of cooking.

The DASH eating plan

Another eating pattern option for people with diabetes is called the DASH eating plan. DASH is an acronym for *Dietary Approaches to Stop Hypertension.* This diet was designed to help lower blood pressure in people with hypertension (or high blood pressure). People with diabetes are at an increased risk for cardiovascular complications, and keeping blood pressure under control may help prevent these complications, so this eating plan may be a good option for some people with diabetes.

The DASH eating plan, similar to the Mediterranean-style eating plan (see the preceding section), promotes eating more fruits and vegetables, whole grains, and legumes, as well as low-fat dairy, poultry, and fish. This eating pattern is relatively high in fiber and nutrients such as potassium, calcium, and magnesium, which may help lower blood pressure.

What kind of foods should you avoid when trying to reduce your blood pressure and protect your heart? The DASH eating plan limits red meat, high-sugar foods (such as sugar-sweetened drinks and sugary desserts), and saturated fat (found in butter, margarine, full-fat dairy products, and high-fat meats). It's also important to limit your intake of foods that are high in sodium.

If you and your dietitian decide that the DASH diet is the right eating pattern for you, you may want to discuss setting a daily sodium intake goal that will help you meet your diabetes and heart-health goals.

Going vegetarian/vegan

Considering a vegetarian or vegan lifestyle? Plant-based eating patterns provide more carbohydrate than other eating patterns, but they can still be an option for people with diabetes. Vegetarian and vegan eating patterns are based on plant foods — such as fruits, vegetables, beans, nuts, seeds, and whole grains — with little to no animal products. The benefit to plant-based eating patterns is that they're rich in fiber, vitamins, and minerals and low in cholesterol and saturated fat, which may reduce the risk of chronic diseases.

Although there hasn't been much research that looks specifically at the effects of vegetarian or vegan diets in people with diabetes, research in the general population has linked following a plant-based eating pattern to a lower risk of obesity, heart disease, cancer, and diabetes.

There are a few different kinds of plant-based eating patterns that vary depending on the type and amount of animal products included. Check out these options to see if any will meet your needs:

>> **Vegan:** A vegan eating plan includes many plant foods, but no animal products at all. People following a vegan diet avoid all meats, poultry, eggs, fish and seafood, dairy, and (in many cases) even honey.

>> **Lacto-vegetarian:** A lacto-vegetarian eating plan includes plant foods and (unlike a vegan eating plan) dairy products such as milk, cheese, and yogurt. People who follow a lacto-vegetarian meal plan also avoid all meats, poultry, eggs, fish, and seafood.

>> **Ovo-lacto vegetarian:** An ovo-lacto vegetarian eating plan includes plant foods, as well as dairy products and eggs. People following this eating pattern still avoid all meats, poultry, fish, and seafood.

Some people choose to be a little more flexible and follow a semi-vegetarian eating pattern, which generally means that their eating pattern is primarily plant-based and they may include dairy, eggs, or even seafood on occasion, but they avoid poultry and red meat. You don't need to follow a strict vegetarian eating pattern to include more fruits, vegetables, and whole grains in your meal plan. Eating vegetarian or vegan dishes for even just a few meals or days per week will help you increase your intake of nutritious plant foods.

Keep in mind that a vegan or vegetarian eating pattern isn't automatically healthy. As with any meal plan or eating pattern, people following a plant-based eating pattern must make nutritious food choices and control their portion sizes. Aim to eat mostly fresh produce, whole grains (rather than refined grain products), beans, nuts, and seeds. Avoid eating a lot of highly processed products and foods that are high in sugar and/or sodium.

WARNING

Meat substitutes, such as tofu, seitan, veggie burgers, and soy-based "meat" or "chicken" products, look like and may taste similar to meat and poultry. You can include these products in your plant-based diet if you choose, but pay attention to the information on the Nutrition Facts label (see Chapter 18). These products can be high in calories, carbohydrate, or sodium.

If you're trying to remove animal products from your diet, or if you're already living a vegan or vegetarian lifestyle and you're wondering if it's compatible with managing diabetes, rest assured. Plant-based diets are an option for people with diabetes as long as they choose nutritious plant foods and control their portions. Ask your dietitian or healthcare provider if a vegan or vegetarian diet is right for you.

A low-carbohydrate eating pattern

Many people believe that a low-carbohydrate diet is the "best" meal planning option for people with diabetes. Although this type of eating pattern may work for some people with diabetes, it's certainly not the only option, and it isn't the right eating pattern for everyone with diabetes.

A low-carbohydrate eating pattern focuses mainly on foods that are higher in protein and nonstarchy vegetables that are low in carbohydrate. People following this eating pattern will primarily eat nonstarchy vegetables — for example, carrots, onions, peppers, broccoli, cauliflower, green beans, and salad greens — and proteins and fats. Meats, poultry, fish and seafood, egg, and dairy can all be included in a low-carbohydrate diet. Highly processed sources of carbohydrate and grain foods, on the other hand, are usually avoided by people following this eating pattern. This generally includes rice, breads, pastas, and sugary foods and drinks.

There is no definition of how many grams of carbohydrate constitute a "low carbohydrate" diet. If you think that a low-carbohydrate eating pattern may be a good fit for you, talk to your dietitian or healthcare provider. He or she can help you find the best way to meet your nutritional needs and set daily carbohydrate goals. (For information on how to keep track of your carbohydrate intake, see Chapter 18.)

REMEMBER

People following a low-carbohydrate eating pattern still benefit from making nutritious food choices. Frequently eating high-fat meats and full-fat dairy products, covering your nonstarchy vegetables in dressing and saturated fat (from butter and margarine), and adding lots of salt to your food isn't good for you in the long run. Even if your blood glucose is well managed, eating a lot of saturated (and trans) fats and sodium can increase your risk of cardiovascular (heart and blood vessel) complications.

The skinny on low-fat diets

A low-fat eating pattern is another option for people with diabetes. This type of eating pattern includes vegetables, fruits, starches, lean proteins, and low-fat dairy products. The best protein options for a low-fat eating pattern are fish and poultry without skin. Limit your intake of excess fat, especially sources of saturated fat (such as butter, margarine, and other hard fats).

Following a low-fat eating pattern may improve heart health when overall calorie intake is also reduced and weight loss occurs. However, in studies, a low-fat diet didn't always improve blood glucose levels or reduce heart disease risk factors. Talk to your dietitian or healthcare provider to determine if this eating pattern can help you achieve your diabetes goals.

TECHNICAL STUFF

According to the American Diabetes Association's position statement "Nutrition Therapy Recommendations for the Management of Adults with Diabetes," a low-fat eating pattern is defined as a total fat intake that is less than 30 percent of a person's total calorie intake and a saturated fat intake that is less than 10 percent of total calorie intake. If you and your dietitian agree that a low-fat eating pattern is right for you, he or she can help you determine how many grams of fat to aim for each day and how to do that.

Glycemic Index and Load

The *glycemic index* (GI) measures how different carbohydrate-containing foods affect blood glucose. The carbohydrate-containing foods are ranked based on how each food's effect on blood glucose compares to that of a standard reference food (pure glucose). A food with a high GI will raise blood glucose levels more than lower-GI foods.

Foods with a GI of 70 or above are considered high-GI foods, while anything with a GI of 55 or under is considered a low-GI food. Medium-GI foods have a GI between 56 and 69. Some examples of relatively low-GI foods include beans, peas, and lentils, many fruits and nonstarchy vegetables, and sweet potatoes, yams, and corn.

REMEMBER

The glycemic index represents the type of carbohydrate in foods, not the amount. The serving sizes and how many grams of carbohydrate are in the foods you're eating are still important. Watch your portions!

Glycemic load (GL) measures the impact that both the *type* and *amount* of carbohydrate in a certain food will have on blood glucose levels. It's calculated by multiplying a food's glycemic index by the amount of carbohydrate in the food/serving. As with the glycemic index, foods with a high GL have a greater impact on blood glucose than lower-GL foods do. Glycemic load may not be a practical tool for everyday meal planning; the glycemic index is more widely used and predictable than glycemic load. (For more information about GI and GL, check out *Glycemic Index Diet For Dummies* by Meri Reffetto [Wiley].)

Both the type and amount of carbohydrate in a food affect blood glucose levels, but studies show that the quantity of carbohydrate in a food generally has a stronger effect on blood glucose than the quality (the GI). This means that the first step toward blood glucose management for most people with diabetes, at least in terms of meal planning, will be some sort of carbohydrate counting/control rather than using the glycemic index. However, the glycemic index (and possibly glycemic load) may be useful tools when used in conjunction with carbohydrate control, for people who are looking to fine-tune their diabetes management efforts.

5

The Part of Tens

IN THIS PART . . .

Explore nutritious snack options and discover how to use snacks to your advantage.

Navigate restaurant menus and get creative with your order to enjoy healthy options.

Chapter **21**

Ten Tips for Smart Snacking

lanning your meals is an important part of successful diabetes management. But what about snacks? Can they be part of a diabetes meal plan?
Absolutely! Snacks can be a great way to curb your appetite and fit more
nutritious foods into your meal plan. Not everyone needs to include snacks in their
diabetes meal plan, but there are several reasons why having a snack or two each
day may be right for you. You may want to consider adding a snack to your meal
plan if you're prone to episodes of low blood glucose (hypoglycemia) or you have
a long stretch between meals.

The key to including snacks in your meal plan is making healthy choices and pay-
ing attention to the amount of carbohydrate you eat at snack time. Even a small
snack can contain a lot of carbohydrate, so be sure to account for that.

This chapter helps you make the most of your snacks. Even if you don't typically
need a snack but you're having one of those days where you need something extra
to munch on, it's important to make healthy choices. We now present ten tips for
better snacks and take a look at some nutritious snack options!

Talk to Your Dietitian

A registered dietitian (RD) or registered dietitian nutritionist (RDN), diabetes educator, or other diabetes care professional will be your go-to resource for all your healthy eating and meal planning needs. It's important to discuss any changes to your eating patterns with your dietitian, and adding snacks to your meal plan is no exception. Before you begin snacking, consult your dietitian to make sure that including a snack in your meal plan is the best option for you. In some cases, your dietitian may suggest including snacks in your meal plan based on your eating habits, physical activity level, or diabetes goals.

If there is a specific reason why you need a snack, share that reason with your dietitian. Maybe your work schedule means you have to wait several hours between lunch and dinner. Or maybe you've noticed that your blood glucose level is low around the same time each day. It's important to discuss this information with your dietitian so he or she can make sure your meal plan meets your needs.

If snacks are included in your meal plan, your dietitian can also help you figure out how many grams of carbohydrate will work for you. Some people may be able to eat about 15 grams of carbohydrate per snack; others may need more or less. If you don't use carbohydrate counting, your dietitian may be able to give you some examples of the kinds of snacks that are right for you.

REMEMBER

Carbohydrate is the nutrient in foods like breads, pastas, grains, fruits, and vegetables that is directly responsible for causing your blood glucose level to rise after eating. It's important for all people with diabetes to be aware of their carbohydrate intake.

Choose Your Snacks Wisely

When it comes to snack foods, people often think of salty or sweet foods like potato chips and dip, pretzels, cookies, and candy. These kinds of snack foods are often high in carbohydrate and may have a lot of added sugar, sodium, and fat. They aren't the best options for most people.

Luckily, there are many nutritious snack options that people with diabetes can enjoy. Think of your snacks as an opportunity to add even more nutrients to your day. Opt for nutritious whole foods — such as nonstarchy vegetables, fresh fruits, nuts (look for nuts that are low in sodium), or low-fat dairy products — over highly processed snacks.

Some light nutritious snack options that contain about 5 grams of carbohydrate or less include

>> 5 baby carrots

>> 5 cherry tomatoes or 1 cup of cucumber slices with 1 tablespoon of ranch dressing

>> 3 celery sticks and 1 tablespoon of peanut butter

>> 1 hard-boiled egg

>> 10 goldfish crackers

>> 1 light string cheese

A few heartier options with about 15–20 grams of carbohydrate include

>> 3 cups of light popcorn

>> 1 small apple

>> ⅓ cup of hummus and 1 cup of raw veggies

>> 5 whole-wheat crackers and 1 light string cheese

>> ½ turkey sandwich (made with 1 slice whole-wheat bread and 2 slices of turkey)

>> ½ peanut butter sandwich (made with 1 slice whole wheat bread and 1 tablespoon of peanut butter)

>> ¼ cup of dried fruit and nut mix

Watch Your Portions

Practicing portion control is an important part of any diabetes meal plan and should extend to any snacks you eat. Eating the right portion sizes for you when you snack is the key to maintaining blood glucose in your target range and avoiding unwanted weight gain.

Make sure you pay attention to the serving size on the Nutrition Facts label when snacking. If you eat double the serving size listed on the label, you're also doubling the amount of calories, carbohydrate, and other nutrients you're consuming.

TIP

Use measuring cups and spoons to verify serving sizes. It's easy to serve yourself a few extra goldfish crackers or an extra tablespoon of peanut butter if you're estimating your servings by sight. Your eyes can be deceiving!

Avoid Mindless Eating

Have you ever curled up on the couch to watch a movie with a big bowl of popcorn or a box of your favorite cookies, and before you even realized it, the bowl or box was empty? Snacking while you're distracted can lead to overeating, especially if a full bag, box, or bowl of food is in front of you.

TIP

Try not to eat in front of the television or computer screen, or while reading or scrolling through your phone. It's even easy to overeat at your desk at work. Here are a few other tips to help you avoid mindless eating:

>> **Focus on chewing each mouthful of food at least ten times before swallowing, and try to pay attention to each bite.** Eating slower may help you realize that you're full sooner.

>> **Enjoy your snacks in a distraction-free environment.** For example, try eating your snacks at your kitchen table or in the break room at work. Taking a few minutes away from your desk or your responsibilities at home to enjoy a snack may even leave you feeling refreshed and ready to get back to your day.

>> **Pay attention to how you feel.** As you're eating, try to pay attention to your body's signals to help you become more aware of when you're full. It can take over 15 minutes after eating for you to feel full.

>> **Don't skip meals.** Try to eat your meals around the same time each day so you won't feel hungry and be tempted to overeat at snack time.

>> **Portion out your snacks instead of eating out of the box or bag.** Place one serving of your snack food in a bowl or on a plate before you eat it. You'll be less tempted to overindulge if you don't have more than one serving in front of you. When you purchase snack foods like crackers, nuts, or dried fruit, try to portion them out and put each serving of the food into a small resealable plastic bag so you can easily grab just the right amount when you need it.

Stock Up on Healthy Options

When you're feeling hungry, it's easy to reach for foods that are less than healthy. You may be tempted at snack time to grab your favorite processed food just because it's quick and familiar, or you may find yourself eating foods from a vending machine at work or a fast-food restaurant just because these foods are convenient. One way to prevent yourself from grabbing these foods is to make sure you always have healthy snack options on hand.

TIP

Make sure you include healthy snacks on your grocery list. Planning your snacks is just as important as planning your meals. Try to select snacks from the perimeter of the grocery store — where you'll find foods like fresh fruit, vegetables, nuts, and low-fat dairy products — rather than the aisles, which are full of processed foods.

Take nutritious snacks with you when you're on the go! If you have a desk at work, store a few nonperishable snacks in a drawer to have on hand. Or keep a serving of crackers or even a healthy granola bar in your purse or in your car for those days when you forget to pack a snack. If you plan ahead and make sure you have healthy foods at your fingertips, you'll be less likely to choose unhealthy snacks.

Be Selfish with Your Snacks

Have you ever bought something for yourself at the grocery store only to realize a few days later that someone else has eaten it? If you have children, a spouse, or a roommate, this scenario probably sounds all too familiar to you.

Sometimes, others can get to the healthy snacks before you do, leaving you with limited options when it's time to eat a snack. Don't be afraid to make sure you have the nutritious foods you need. Stock up on your favorite healthy snack foods so you have enough for the whole family — everyone can benefit from snacking healthier! At work, don't be shy about labeling any snacks you leave in the break room so you'll have them when you need them.

Snacks for Low Blood Glucose

If you're prone to low blood glucose (hypoglycemia), then your dietitian may have already recommended that you include snacks in your meal plan to prevent your blood glucose levels from dropping too low (a blood glucose reading below 70 mg/dL). But what can you eat *during* an episode of hypoglycemia to bring your blood glucose levels back to the normal range?

Many people find it convenient to carry glucose tablets or gels with them for treating lows. But if you start feeling the symptoms of low blood glucose unexpectedly — for example, shakiness, dizziness, hunger/nausea, sweating, chills, weakness, and mood swings — and don't have glucose on hand, you need to know what you can eat or drink. Your normal snacks may not be appropriate for treating low blood glucose, especially if they contain protein or fat (which may increase the time it takes for the carbohydrate to raise your blood glucose and provide unnecessary calories). Instead, you'll want to consume 15–20 grams of simple carbohydrate, which are digested quickly. Good options with about 15 grams of carbohydrate include

>> 2 tablespoons of raisins

>> 4 or 5 saltine crackers

>> 1 tablespoon of sugar, honey, or corn syrup

>> ½ cup of juice or regular soda (not diet)

REMEMBER

If you suspect that your blood glucose is low, first use a blood glucose meter to confirm low blood glucose. Once confirmed, follow these steps to treat the low:

1. Consume 15–20 grams of simple carbohydrate.

2. Recheck your blood glucose after 15 minutes.

3. Repeat this process until your blood glucose level returns to normal.

After an episode of low blood glucose, you'll want to eat a small, healthy snack if your next meal is still a few hours away.

Snack before a Big Meal or Event

Holidays, birthdays, and big family events can be tricky situations for people with diabetes. Events like these often feature less than healthy foods in large quantities, making it very easy to overindulge, especially if you arrive to the party on an empty stomach. Having a light, healthy snack — just enough to prevent you from feeling starved — before going to a big party may help satisfy your hunger so you're less tempted to eat too much at the party and you can make food choices with a clear head. If you're not starving, you may be more inclined to take a few moments and consider the healthiest options available to you when you arrive at the event.

Think Outside the Box

Snacks don't have to be boring just because you have diabetes. Try to avoid processed foods that are high in calories, carbohydrate, and sodium, but you don't have to snack on celery sticks or a rice cakes every day. Get creative! If you have leftovers from dinner the night before, portion out a small amount (based on the snack guidelines you discuss with your dietitian) and enjoy!

You can also use diabetes-friendly recipes, like the recipes in this book, to your advantage. Light and tasty appetizers and nonstarchy vegetable side dishes can be excellent snacks when eaten in the right portion size. Try the Cheesy Tortilla Wedges, Guacamole, or Cucumber Pâté, and other tasty appetizers from Chapter 10. Or spice up your snacks with veggie dishes like Carrots Marsala or Snow Peas with Sesame Seeds (find these recipes in Chapter 12). You can make diabetes-friendly dishes as a snack for the whole family, or enjoy one serving and save the rest to snack on later in the week. Just make sure you watch your portion sizes!

Don't Deprive Yourself

It's important to choose healthy snack options if you have diabetes. But if there is a snack food that you absolutely love, you don't have to cut it out of your life completely just because it's a little too high in calories or carbohydrate. You don't have to deprive yourself of the foods you love because you have diabetes. Adjusting to a diabetes meal plan can sometimes feel restricting or overwhelming, so it's important to find ways to enjoy the foods you love. Indulging in your favorite foods now and then can certainly fit into a healthy meal plan. Talk to your dietitian or provider if you're struggling with cravings and food choices.

» Asking your server the right questions

» Getting creative with the menu

» Navigating fast-food menus

Chapter 22

Ten Strategies for Healthier Restaurant Meals

Cooking healthy meals is an essential skill to make good diabetes management easier. But there are days when eating at home just isn't in the cards. Maybe you're planning to go out to dinner with a group of friends, or you're working late one evening and you won't have the time or energy to cook when you get home. Or maybe you'd just like to enjoy a meal at your favorite restaurant. It's important to know how to navigate restaurant menus for occasions like these.

Dining out can be challenging for people with diabetes. When you prepare a healthy meal at home, you're in the driver's seat; you have complete control over the ingredients and cooking methods you use and the amount of food you serve yourself. You don't have the same amount of control when you order food at a restaurant. But don't worry! With a little advance planning and creative thinking, you can find a dish to fit your meal plan on almost any restaurant menu. In this chapter, we explore some tips and techniques to help you find the find the healthiest options when eating out.

Research Your Restaurant

Believe it or not, you can begin strategizing for your healthy restaurant meal before you even arrive at the restaurant. Take a few minutes before heading out the door to think about the restaurants in your area and select one that will make it easy for you to enjoy a healthy meal.

TIP

If you're not sure what kind of food a restaurant offers, call the restaurant or see if its menu is available online. The Internet is a helpful resource when you're trying to plan restaurant meals — take advantage of it! Many restaurants now provide their full menu online, and most even include nutrition information.

Ideally, you'll want to look for a restaurant that offers a variety of different dishes featuring nutritious ingredients such as nonstarchy vegetables, whole grains, and lean proteins. If the restaurant you choose has nutrition information for its dishes available online, you're one step ahead of the game! You can use this information to figure out exactly how different menu items will fit into your meal plan. It may be a good idea to identify a few options that will work for you before you leave home; that way, you'll be less tempted to order unhealthy menu items when you get to the restaurant.

Ask Your Server

Even if you're able to research the restaurant's menu beforehand, you may have questions about the menu when you arrive. A dish may sound healthy on the menu, but there can be hidden sources of fat and calories in the dish that aren't mentioned in the description of the item. Don't be afraid to ask your server exactly what's in the dish and how it's prepared. Your server may not know all the ingredients or the cooking method offhand, but he or she can check with the chef.

Knowing what goes into the dish you're about to eat will give you a better understanding of how that dish will fit into your diabetes meal plan. If it sounds healthy on the menu, but it's cooked in butter or has a lot of added sodium, you may want to look for another option. Communication with your server is important. If you're having trouble finding good choices on the menu, he or she may be able to steer you in the right direction.

Make Special Requests

If you find a dish on the menu that sounds very appealing but has some less-than-healthy ingredients, feel free to make special requests and ask about substitutions. A few small changes to a dish can make all the difference when it comes to eating healthy, and most restaurants will be happy to accommodate your needs.

If your dish comes with a choice of side items, look for the healthiest options available. That may mean choosing brown rice over white or fried rice, or steamed vegetables instead of mac and cheese. If you have more than one choice, why not double up on nonstarchy vegetables such as green beans, broccoli, cauliflower, asparagus, Brussels sprouts, or a side salad. Even if the menu doesn't offer a choice of sides, you can request to replace starchy sides like fries, potatoes, and rice with healthier options.

Many restaurant dishes are made with healthy ingredients but are cooked in a lot of fat or are topped with high-calorie sauces. Request that the chef leave any heavy sauce off your dish. Or ask the server if a dish can be steamed, grilled, or sautéed in a small amount of olive oil instead of fried or cooked in butter. If you're watching your sodium intake, ask if your meal can be prepared without added salt.

REMEMBER

Don't forget about condiments! Many condiments are sources of fat and carbohydrate. Request mustard on your burger instead of mayonnaise, or skip the dipping cups of barbecue sauce or ranch dressing. Ask your server if the restaurant has low-fat salad dressings that they can substitute for the full-fat version on your salad.

Be respectful of your server, but don't be shy about asking questions and making special requests. Be direct and polite and the restaurant should be able to accommodate your needs.

Helpful Substitutions

Swapping out some of the less-healthy ingredients in a dish for more nutritious options is a great way to enjoy the menu item you're craving without disrupting your meal plan. There are a few common restaurant foods and ingredients that you'll want to request substitutions for whenever you can. Here are a few common substitutions to get you started:

Instead of . . .	Try . . .
Alfredo sauce	Marinara sauce
Cheese and/or bacon (on sandwiches)	Extra fresh vegetables
Cream-based soup	Clear broth soup
Flour tortillas	Corn or whole-wheat tortillas
Fried chicken strips	Chicken kabobs or satay
Fried mozzarella sticks	Caprese (mozzarella and tomato) salad
Fried rice	Steamed brown rice
Heavy sauces	Sautéed mushrooms or onions
Mayonnaise	Mustard
Meat pizza	Veggie pizza
Pan, deep-dish, or stuffed-crust pizza	Thin-crust pizza
Refried beans	Black beans
Sour cream	Salsa
Tempura meat or vegetables	Steamed or grilled meat or vegetables

Skip the Extras

Even if you order a nutritious restaurant dish that fits into your meal plan, it can be easy to get off track when the free bread basket or chips and salsa arrive at the table. These items can contribute a significant amount of extra calories or carbohydrate to your meal. If you have the self-control to have just a bite of bread or a few chips, that's fine. If not, you may want to skip these foods altogether and ask your server not to bring them to the table.

Appetizers are another source of extra calories that you may want to avoid. If you're really craving a certain appetizer, try to split it with others at the table so you only eat a small portion. Make sure you account for it in your meal plan. If you're very hungry when you arrive at the restaurant, try ordering a side salad with low-fat dressing instead of ordering an appetizer or reaching for the bread basket.

Don't Drink Your Calories

It can be tempting to order a regular soda, sweetened iced tea, or maybe even a cocktail with your dish, but these drinks can add a lot of calories and carbohydrate to your meal (which is likely already higher in calories than the meals you cook at home). Save those calories for the food on your plate. If you skip that 120-calorie serving of soda, you may have room in your meal plan to add an extra serving of nonstarchy vegetables to your plate; it's the more satisfying and nutritious option. Remember that mixers in alcoholic beverages (besides diet soda) generally contain carbohydrate and calories as well.

REMEMBER

Try to stick with zero-calorie beverages when you eat out. Water is always a great choice, but you can try diet soda, sparkling water, unsweetened tea, or black coffee.

Take Half Home

Another key aspect of healthy restaurant eating is portion control. Restaurants today often serve customers *huge* portions of food, much more than the average person needs to eat. It's up to you to make sure you don't overeat. This is especially important if you're indulging in a less-healthy menu item — but the calories and carbohydrate still add up if you eat a large portion of a healthier dish.

TIP

If you're concerned about the portion size of your meal, ask for a take-home container and pack up half of the food on your plate before you begin eating. You'll be less likely to overeat if you have an appropriate portion of food in front of you. Out of sight, out of mind. Take the leftovers home and enjoy them for lunch or dinner the next day!

Get Creative with the Menu

When it comes to healthy restaurant eating, sometimes it's helpful to think outside the box. Don't feel pressure to order an entrée for yourself just because that's what other people may be doing. Get creative with the menu! You may be able to build yourself a healthier meal using different menu options.

For people trying to reduce their portion sizes, sharing an entrée (or even just an appetizer) with a friend or loved one is an option. Or you can choose a few healthy side dishes as your main dish. Believe it or not, the side dishes are sometimes the most nutritious items on a menu. Most sit-down restaurants offer at least one or two nonstarchy vegetable side dishes, and in some restaurants you may find beans, whole grains, or even lentils in the list of sides. And portion sizes for side dishes are generally small. Try selecting one or two healthy side options and maybe pairing them with a small salad or broth-based soup as your meal.

Another idea for creating a healthy meal is to add extra nonstarchy vegetables to a dish. Add a side salad with light dressing to an entrée, for example, or ask to add extra fresh vegetables to a sandwich, wrap, or burger. Extra nonstarchy vegetables can add nutrients to your meal and may fill you up so you eat less of the other items on your plate. These are just a few ideas — don't be afraid to take advantage of different menu option to create a meal that's right for you.

Order Takeout before You're Hungry

As with any restaurant meal, it's important to make healthy food choices and watch your portions sizes when ordering takeout from a restaurant. But ordering takeout gives you added advantage: You can order your food *before* you're hungry. It's easier to choose nutritious foods and avoid overeating if you're not starving when you order. If you know you'll be ordering takeout, make a conscious effort to choose and order your food before you start feeling hungry. Some restaurants may even let you order a few hours in advance. Lock in your order early so you won't be tempted by unhealthy options when you're hungry later on.

Choose Fast Foods Wisely

Eating at fast-food restaurants can be particularly challenging for people with diabetes, so you may want to avoid fast-food restaurants when you can. But fast food may be a reality of your fast-paced lifestyle. There will be days when you're extremely busy or you're traveling and fast food seems like your only option. If you find yourself in this situation, here are a few tips that can help you make the healthiest possible choices:

>> Order regular-size or "junior" sandwiches from the menu rather than "double" or "deluxe" items, which are often much larger.

>> Avoid high-fat sandwich toppings like bacon, cheese, mayonnaise, and barbecue sauce. Opt instead for extra veggies and mustard.

>> Opt for grilled or broiled fish and chicken instead of fried proteins and beef. They're leaner.

>> Avoid meal deals. They may seem like a bargain because you get more food for less, but what you're really getting is large portions of fried foods and sugary beverages.

>> Substitute a side salad or fresh fruit for fries if possible.

>> Go bunless. Removing half or all of the bun from your sandwich can save you several grams of carbohydrate.

>> Choose water, diet soda, unsweetened tea, or black coffee as your beverage.

>> Remember that you can make special requests when ordering fast food, too! Don't be afraid to ask the restaurant to accommodate your needs. Just be aware that it may take a few extra minutes for them to prepare a special order.

>> If you find a healthy order that works for you at your favorite fast-food restaurant, remember it so you can easily order it again when you need to.

Appendix

Food Lists

The food lists and information presented in this appendix comes directly from the booklet *Choose Your Foods: Food Lists for Diabetes,* published by the American Diabetes Association and the Academy of Nutrition and Dietetics. These food lists group together foods that have about the same amount of carbohydrate, protein, fat, and calories, and the lists are used by people with diabetes who plan their meals with food choices/exchanges. The term *choice* (formerly *exchange*) is used to describe a certain quantity of food within a group of similar foods.

The first step for people with diabetes using food choices/exchanges to plan their meals is to meet with a registered dietitian (RD) or registered dietitian nutritionist (RDN). A dietitian will help you select the number of choices from each food list that is right for you at each meal (and snack, if snacks are included in your meal plan). The number of choices from each list that you eat will be based on your food preference, lifestyle, diabetes goals, and individual needs.

The Food Lists

The following chart shows the amount of nutrients in one choice from each list.

Food List	Carbohydrate (grams)	Protein (grams)	Fat (grams)	Calories
Carbohydrates				
Starch: breads; cereals; grains and pasta; starchy vegetables; crackers and snacks; and beans, peas, and lentils	15	3	1	80
Fruits	15	—	—	60
Milk and Milk Substitutes				
Fat-free, low-fat (1%)	12	8	0–3	100
Reduced-fat (2%)	12	8	5	120
Whole	12	8	8	160

(continued)

Food List	Carbohydrate (grams)	Protein (grams)	Fat (grams)	Calories
Nonstarchy vegetables	5	2	—	25
Sweets, desserts, and other carbohydrates	15	Varies	Varies	Varies
Proteins				
Lean	—	7	2	45
Medium-fat	—	7	5	75
High-fat	—	7	8	100
Plant-based	Varies	7	Varies	Varies
Fats	—	—	5	45
Alcohol (1 alcohol equivalent)	Varies	—	—	100

Starch

One starch choice has 15 grams of carbohydrate, 3 grams of protein, 1 gram of fat, and 80 calories.

Bread

Food	Serving Size
Bagel	¼ large bagel (1 oz.)
Biscuit*	1 biscuit (2½ inches across)
Breads, loaf-type: white, whole-grain, French, Italian, pumpernickel, rye, sourdough, unfrosted raisin or cinnamon	1 slice (1 oz.)
Breads, loaf-type: reduced-calorie, light**	2 slices (1½ oz.)
Breads, flat-type, chapatti	1 oz.
Breads, flat-type, ciabatta	1 oz.
Breads, flat-type, naan	3¼-inch square (1 oz.)
Breads, flat-type, pita (6 inches across)	½ pita
Breads, flat-type, roti	1 oz.

Food	Serving Size
Breads, flat-type, sandwich flat buns, whole-wheat**	1 bun, including top and bottom (1½ oz.)
Breads, flat-type, taco shell*	2 taco shells (each 5 inches across)
Breads, flat-type, tortilla, corn	1 small tortilla (6 inches across)
Breads, flat-type, tortilla, flour (white or whole-wheat)	1 small tortilla (6 inches across) or ⅓ large tortilla (10 inches across)
Cornbread	1¾-inch cube (1½ oz.)
English muffin	½ muffin
Hot dog bun or hamburger bun	½ bun (¾ oz.)
Pancake	1 pancake (4 inches across, ¼ inch thick)
Roll, plain	1 small roll (1 oz.)
Stuffing, bread*	⅓ cup
Waffle	1 waffle (4-inch square or 4 inches across)

*Extra fat
**Good source of fiber

Cereals

Food	Serving Size
Bran cereal (twigs, buds, or flakes)**	½ cup
Cooked cereals (oats, oatmeal)	½ cup
Granola cereal	¼ cup
Grits, cooked	½ cup
Muesli	¼ cup
Puffed cereal	1½ cups
Shredded wheat, plain	½ cup
Sugar-coated cereal	½ cup
Unsweetened, ready-to-eat cereal	¾ cup

**Good source of fiber

Grains (Including Pasta and Rice)

Food	Serving Size
Barley	⅓ cup
Bran, dry, oat*	¼ cup
Bran, dry, wheat*	½ cup
Bulgur*	½ cup
Couscous	⅓ cup
Kasha	½ cup
Millet	⅓ cup
Pasta, white or whole-wheat (all shapes and sizes)	⅓ cup
Polenta	⅓ cup
Quinoa, all colors	⅓ cup
Rice, white, brown, and other colors and types	⅓ cup
Tabbouleh (tabouli), prepared	½ cup
Wheat germ, dry	3 Tablespoon
Wild rice	½ cup

Note: *Unless otherwise indicated, serving sizes listed are for cooked grains.*
Good source of fiber

Starchy Vegetables

Food	Serving Size
Breadfruit	¼ cup
Cassava or dasheen	⅓ cup
Corn	½ cup
Corn on cob	4- to 4½-inch piece (½ large cob)
Hominy*	¾ cup
Mixed vegetables with corn or peas*	1 cup
Marinara, pasta, or spaghetti sauce	½ cup
Parsnips*	½ cup

Food	Serving Size
Peas, green*	½ cup
Plantain	⅓ cup
Potato, baked with skin	¼ large potato (3 oz.)
Potato, boiled, all kinds	½ cup or ½ medium potato (3 oz.)
Potato, mashed, with milk and fat**	½ cup
Potato, french-fried (oven-baked)***	1 cup (2 oz.)
Pumpkin puree, canned, no sugar added*	¾ cup
Squash, winter (acorn, butternut)*	1 cup
Succotash*	½ cup
Yam or sweet potato, plain	½ cup (3½ oz.)

Note: All the serving sizes for starchy vegetables on this list are for cooked vegetables.
*Good source of fiber
**Extra fat
***Restaurant-style French fries are on the Fast Foods list, later in this appendix.

Crackers and Snacks

Food	Serving Size
Crackers, animal	8 crackers
Crackers, crispbread*	2–5 pieces (¾ oz.)
Crackers, graham, 2½-inch square	3 squares
Crackers, nut and rice	10 crackers
Crackers, oyster	20 crackers
Crackers, round, butter-type**	6 crackers
Crackers, saltine-type	6 crackers
Crackers, sandwich-style, cheese or peanut butter filling**	3 crackers
Crackers, whole-wheat, baked	5 regular 1½-inch squares or 10 thins (¾ oz.)
Granola or snack bar	1 bar (¾ oz.)
Matzoh, all shapes and sizes	¾ oz.

(continued)

(continued)

Food	Serving Size
Melba toast	4 pieces (each about 2 by 4 inches)
Popcorn, no fat added*	3 cups
Popcorn, with butter added***	3 cups
Pretzels	¾ oz.
Rice cakes	2 cakes (4 inches across)
Snack chips, baked (potato, pita)	About 8 chips (¾ oz.)
Snack chips, regular (tortilla, potato)***	About 13 chips (1 oz.)

Note: For other snacks, see the Sweets, Desserts, and Other Carbohydrates list, later in this appendix.

Note: Some snacks are high in fat. Always check food labels.

Good source of fiber

**Extra fat, counts as 1 starch choice + 1 fat choice (1 starch choice plus 5 grams of fat)*

***Extra fat, counts as 1 starch choice + 2 fat choices (1 starch choice plus 10 grams of fat)*

Beans, Peas, and Lentils

Food	Serving Size
Baked beans, canned*	⅓ cup
Beans (black, garbanzo, kidney, lima, navy, pinto, white), cooked or canned, drained and rinsed*	½ cup
Lentils (any color), cooked*	½ cup
Peas (black-eyed and split), cooked or canned, drained and rinsed*	½ cup
Refried beans, canned*/**	½ cup

Note: The choices on this list count as 1 starch choice + 1 lean protein choice.

Note: Beans, lentils, and peas are also found on the Protein list, later in this appendix.

Good source of fiber

**High in sodium*

Fruits

One fruit choice has 15 grams of carbohydrate and 60 calories.

Fruits

Food	Serving Size
Apple, unpeeled	1 small apple (4 oz.)
Apples, dried	4 rings
Applesauce, unsweetened	½ cup
Apricots, canned	½ cup
Apricots, dried	8 apricot halves
Apricots, fresh	4 apricots (5½ oz. total)
Banana	1 extra-small banana, about 4 inches long (4 oz.)
Blackberries*	1 cup
Blueberries	¾ cup
Cantaloupe	1 cup diced
Cherries, sweet, canned	½ cup
Cherries, sweet, fresh	12 cherries (3½ oz.)
Dates	3 small (deglet noor) dates or 1 large (medjool) date
Dried fruits (blueberries, cherries, cranberries, mixed fruit, raisins)	2 tablespoons
Figs, dried	3 small figs
Figs, fresh*	1½ large or 2 medium figs (3½ oz. total)
Fruit cocktail	½ cup
Grapefruit, fresh	½ large grapefruit (5½ oz.)
Grapefruit, sections, canned	¾ cup
Grapes	17 small grapes (3 oz. total)
Guava*	2 small guava (2½ oz. total)
Honeydew melon	1 cup diced
Kiwi	½ cup sliced
Loquat	¾ cup cubed
Mandarin oranges, canned	¾ cup
Mango	½ small mango (5½ oz.) or ½ cup

(continued)

(continued)

Food	Serving Size
Nectarine	1 medium nectarine (5½ oz.)
Orange*	1 medium orange (6½ oz.)
Papaya	½ papaya (8 oz.) or 1 cup cubed
Peaches, canned	½ cup
Peaches, fresh	1 medium peach (6 oz.)
Pears, canned	½ cup
Pears, fresh*	½ large pear (4 oz.)
Pineapple, canned	½ cup
Pineapple, fresh	¾ cup
Plantain, extra-ripe (black), raw	¼ plantain (2¼ oz.)
Plums, canned	½ cup
Plums, dried (prunes)	3 prunes
Plums, fresh	2 small plums (5 oz. total)
Pomegranate seeds (arils)	½ cup
Raspberries*	1 cup
Strawberries*	1¼ cup whole berries
Tangerine	1 large tangerine (6 oz.)
Watermelon	1¼ cups diced

Note: *The weights listed include skin, core, seeds, and rind.*
*= Good source of fiber

Fruit Juice

Food	Serving Size
Apple juice/cider	½ cup
Fruit juice blends, 100% juice	⅓ cup
Grape juice	⅓ cup
Grapefruit juice	½ cup
Orange juice	½ cup

Food	Serving Size
Pineapple juice	½ cup
Pomegranate juice	½ cup
Prune juice	⅓ cup

Milk and Milk Substitutes

One carbohydrate choice has 15 grams of carbohydrate and about 70 calories. One fat choice has 5 grams of fat and 45 calories.

Milk and Yogurts

Food	Serving Size	Choices per Serving
Fat-free (skim) or low-fat (1%) milk, buttermilk, acidophilus milk, lactose-free milk	1 cup	1 fat-free milk
Fat-free (skim) or low-fat (1%) evaporated milk	½ cup	1 fat-free milk
Fat-free (skim) or low-fat (1%) yogurt, plain or Greek; may be sweetened with an artificial sweetener	⅓ cup (6 oz.)	1 fat-free milk
Fat-free (skim) or low-fat (1%) chocolate milk	1 cup	1 fat-free milk + 1 carbohydrate
Reduced-fat (2%) milk, acidophilus milk, kefir, lactose-free milk	1 cup	1 reduced-fat milk
Reduced-fat (2%) yogurt, plain	⅓ cup (6 oz.)	1 reduced-fat milk
Whole milk, buttermilk, goat's milk	1 cup	1 whole milk
Whole evaporated milk	½ cup	1 whole milk
Whole yogurt, plain	1 cup (8 oz.)	1 whole milk
Whole chocolate milk	1 cup	1 whole milk + 1 carbohydrate

Other Milk Foods and Milk Substitutes

Food	Serving Size	Choices per Serving
Eggnog		
fat-free	⅓ cup	1 carbohydrate
low-fat	⅓ cup	1 carbohydrate + ½ fat
whole milk	⅓ cup	1 carbohydrate + 1 fat
Rice drink		
plain, fat-free	1 cup	1 carbohydrate
flavored, low-fat	1 cup	2 carbohydrates
Soy milk		
light or low-fat, plain	1 cup	½ carbohydrate + ½ fat
regular, plain	1 cup	½ carbohydrate + 1 fat
Yogurt with fruit, low-fat	⅓ cup (6 oz.)	1 fat-free milk + 1 carbohydrate

Note: *Unsweetened nut milks (such as almond milk and coconut milk) are on the Fats list.*

Nonstarchy Vegetables

One nonstarchy vegetable choice (½ cup cooked or 1 cup raw) has 5 grams of carbohydrate, 2 grams of protein, 0 grams of fat, and 25 calories.

Nonstarchy Vegetables

Amaranth leaves (Chinese spinach)	Beets
Artichoke	Broccoli
Artichoke hearts (no oil)	Broccoli slaw, packaged, no dressing
Asparagus	Brussels sprouts*
Baby corn	Cabbage (green, red, bok choy, Chinese)
Bamboo shoots	Carrots*
Bean sprouts (alfalfa, mung, soybean)	Cauliflower
Beans (green, wax, Italian, yard-long beans)	Celery

Chayote	Okra
Coleslaw, packaged, no dressing	Onions
Cucumber	Pea pods
Daikon	Peppers (all varieties)
Eggplant	Radishes
Fennel	Rutabaga
Gourds (bitter, bottle, luffa, bitter melon)	Sauerkraut, drained and rinsed**
Green onions or scallions	Spinach
Greens (collard, dandelion, mustard, purslane, turnip)	Squash, summer varieties (yellow, pattypan, crookneck, zucchini)
Hearts of palm	Sugar snap peas
Jicama*	Swiss chard
Kale	Tomato
Kohlrabi	Tomatoes, canned
Leeks	Tomato sauce (unsweetened)**
Mixed vegetables (without starchy vegetables, legumes, or pasta)	Tomato/vegetable juice
	Turnips
Mushrooms, all kinds, fresh	Water chestnuts

*Good source of fiber
**High in sodium

Sweets, Desserts, and Other Carbohydrates

One carbohydrate choice has 15 grams of carbohydrate and about 70 calories. One fat choice has 5 grams of fat and 45 calories.

Beverages, Soda, and Sports Drinks

Food	Serving Size	Choices per Serving
Cranberry juice cocktail	½ cup	1 carbohydrate
Fruit drink or lemonade	1 cup (8 oz.)	2 carbohydrates

(continued)

(continued)

Food	Serving Size	Choices per Serving
Hot chocolate, regular	1 envelope (2 tablespoons or ¾ oz.) added to 8 oz. water	1 carbohydrate
Soft drink (soda), regular	1 can (12 oz.)	2½ carbohydrates
Sports drink (fluid replacement type)	1 cup (8 oz.)	1 carbohydrate

Brownies, Cake, Cookies, Gelatin, Pie, and Pudding

Food	Serving Size	Choices per Serving
Biscotti	1 oz.	1 carbohydrate + 1 fat
Brownie, small, unfrosted	1¼-inch square, ⅞-inch high (about 1 oz.)	1 carbohydrate + 1 fat
Cake, angel food, unfrosted	$\frac{1}{12}$ of cake (about 2 oz.)	2 carbohydrates
Cake, frosted	2-inch square (about 2 oz.)	2 carbohydrates + 1 fat
Cake, unfrosted	2-inch square (about 1 oz.)	1 carbohydrate + 1 fat
Cookies, 100-calorie pack	1 oz.	1 carbohydrate + ½ fat
Cookies, chocolate chip	2 cookies, 2¼ inches across	1 carbohydrate + 2 fats
Cookies, gingersnaps	3 small cookies, 1½ inches across	1 carbohydrate
Cookies, large	1 cookie, 6 inches across (about 3 oz.)	4 carbohydrates + 3 fats
Cookies, sandwich cookies with crème filling	2 small cookies (about ⅔ oz.)	1 carbohydrate + 1 fat
Cookies, sugar-free	1 large or 3 small cookies (¾–1 oz.)	1 carbohydrate + 1–2 fats
Cookies, vanilla wafer	5 cookies	1 carbohydrate + 1 fat
Cupcake, frosted	1 small cupcake (about 1¾ oz.)	2 carbohydrates + 1–1½ fats
Flan	½ cup	2½ carbohydrates + 1 fat
Fruit cobbler	½ cup (3½ oz.)	3 carbohydrates + 1 fat
Gelatin, regular	½ cup	1 carbohydrate
Pie, commercially prepared fruit, 2 crusts	⅙ of 8-inch pie	3 carbohydrates + 2 fats
Pie, pumpkin or custard	⅛ of 8-inch pie	1½ carbohydrates + 1½ fats

Food	Serving Size	Choices per Serving
Pudding, regular (made with reduced-fat milk)	½ cup	2 carbohydrates
Pudding, sugar-free or sugar- and fat-free (made with fat-free milk)	½ cup	1 carbohydrate

Candy, Spreads, Sweets, Sweeteners, Syrups, and Toppings

Food	Serving Size	Choices per Serving
Blended sweeteners (mixtures of artificial sweeteners and sugar)	1½ tablespoons	1 carbohydrate
Candy, chocolate, dark or milk type	1 oz.	1 carbohydrate + 2 fats
Candy, chocolate "kisses"	5 pieces	1 carbohydrate + 1 fat
Candy, hard	3 pieces	1 carbohydrate
Coffee creamer, nondairy type, powdered, flavored	4 teaspoons	½ carbohydrate + ½ fat
Coffee creamer, nondairy type, liquid, flavored	2 tablespoons	1 carbohydrate
Fruit snacks, chewy (pureed fruit concentrate)	1 roll (¾ oz.)	1 carbohydrate
Fruit spreads, 100% fruit	1½ tablespoons	1 carbohydrate
Honey	1 tablespoon	1 carbohydrate
Jam or jelly, regular	1 tablespoon	1 carbohydrate
Sugar	1 tablespoon	1 carbohydrate
Syrup, chocolate	2 tablespoons	2 carbohydrates
Syrup, light (pancake-type)	2 tablespoons	1 carbohydrate
Syrup, regular (pancake-type)	1 tablespoon	1 carbohydrate

Condiments and Sauces

Food	Serving Size	Choices per Serving
Barbecue sauce	3 tablespoons	1 carbohydrate
Cranberry sauce, jellied	¼ cup	1½ carbohydrates
Curry sauce*	1 oz.	1 carbohydrate + 1 fat
Gravy, canned or bottled*	½ cup	½ carbohydrate + ½ fat

(continued)

(continued)

Food	Serving Size	Choices per Serving
Hoisin sauce	1 tablespoon	½ carbohydrate
Marinade	1 tablespoon	½ carbohydrate
Plum sauce	1 tablespoon	½ carbohydrate
Salad dressing, fat-free, cream-based	3 tablespoons	1 carbohydrate
Sweet-and-sour sauce	3 tablespoons	1 carbohydrate

Note: You can also check the Fats list and Free Foods list for other condiments.
*High in sodium

Doughnuts, Muffins, Pastries, and Sweet Breads

Food	Serving Size	Choices per Serving
Banana nut bread	1-inch slice (2 oz.)	2 carbohydrates + 1 fat
Doughnut, cake, plain	1 medium doughnut (1½ oz.)	1½ carbohydrates + 2 fats
Doughnut, hole	2 holes (1 oz.)	1 carbohydrate + 1 fat
Doughnut, yeast-type, glazed	1 doughnut, 3¾ inches across (2 oz.)	2 carbohydrates + 2 fats
Muffin, regular	1 muffin (4 oz.)	4 carbohydrates + 2½ fats
Muffin, lower-fat	1 muffin (4 oz.)	4 carbohydrates + ½ fat
Scone	1 scone (4 oz.)	4 carbohydrates + 3 fats
Sweet roll or Danish	1 pastry (2½ oz.)	2½ carbohydrates + 2 fats

Frozen Bars, Frozen Desserts, Frozen Yogurt, and Ice Cream

Food	Serving Size	Choices per Serving
Frozen pops	1	½ carbohydrate
Fruit juice bars, frozen, 100% juice	1 bar (3 oz.)	1 carbohydrate
Ice cream, fat-free	½ cup	1½ carbohydrates
Ice cream, light	½ cup	1 carbohydrate + 1 fat
Ice cream, no-sugar-added	½ cup	1 carbohydrate + 1 fat
Ice cream, regular	½ cup	1 carbohydrate + 2 fats
Sherbet, sorbet	½ cup	2 carbohydrates

Food	Serving Size	Choices per Serving
Yogurt, frozen, fat-free	⅓ cup	1 carbohydrate
Yogurt, frozen, regular	½ cup	1 carbohydrate + 0–1 fat
Yogurt, frozen, Greek, lower-fat or fat-free	½ cup	1½ carbohydrates

Protein

Meat, fish, poultry, cheese, eggs, and plant-based foods are all sources of protein and have varying amounts of fat. Foods from this list are divided into four groups based on the amount of fat they contain: lean protein, medium-fat protein, high-fat protein, and plant-based protein.

Lean protein

One lean protein choice has 0 grams of carbohydrate, 7 grams of protein, 2 grams of fat, and 45 calories.

Note: The serving size for meat, fish, poultry, or hard cheeses is usually 1 ounce.

Lean Protein

Food	Serving Size
Beef: ground (90% or higher lean/10% or lower fat); select or choice grades trimmed of fat: roast (chuck, round, rump, sirloin), steak (cubed, flank, porterhouse, T-bone), tenderloin	1 oz.
Beef jerky*	½ oz.
Cheeses with 3 grams of fat or less per ounce	1 oz.
Curd-style cheeses: cottage-type (all kinds), ricotta (fat-free or light)	¼ cup (2 oz.)
Egg substitutes, plain	¼ cup
Egg whites	2
Fish, fresh or frozen, such as catfish, cod, flounder, haddock, halibut, orange roughy, tilapia, trout	1 oz.
Fish, salmon, fresh or canned	1 oz.

(continued)

Food	Serving Size
Fish, sardines, canned	2 small sardines
Fish, tuna, fresh or canned in water or oil and drained	1 oz.
Fish, smoked: herring or salmon (lox)*	1 oz.
Game: buffalo, ostrich, rabbit, venison	1 oz.
Hot dog with 3 grams of fat or less per ounce*/**	1 hot dog (1¾ oz.)
Lamb: chop, leg, or roast	1 oz.
Organ meats: heart, kidney, liver***	1 oz.
Oysters, fresh or frozen	6 medium oysters
Pork, lean, Canadian bacon*	1 oz.
Pork, lean, ham*	1 oz.
Pork, lean, rib or loin chop/roast, tenderloin	1 oz.
Poultry, without skin: chicken, Cornish hen, domestic duck or goose (well drained of fat), turkey, lean ground turkey or chicken	1 oz.
Processed sandwich meats with 3 grams of fat or less per ounce: chipped beef, thin-sliced deli meats, turkey ham, turkey pastrami*	1 oz.
Sausage with 3 grams of fat or less per ounce*	1 oz.
Shellfish: clams, crab, imitation shellfish, lobster, scallops, shrimp	1 oz.
Veal: cutlet (no breading), loin chop, roast	1 oz.

High in sodium (based on the sodium content of a typical 3-ounce serving of meat, unless 1 ounce or 2 ounces is the normal serving size
**May contain carbohydrate*
***May be high in cholesterol*

Medium-fat protein

One medium–fat protein choice has 0 grams of carbohydrate, 7 grams of protein, 5 grams of fat, and 75 calories.

Note: The serving size for meat, fish, poultry, or hard cheeses is usually 1 ounce.

Medium-Fat Protein

Food	Serving Size
Beef trimmed of visible fat: ground beef (85% or lower lean/15% or higher fat), corned beef, meatloaf, prime cuts of beef (rib roast), short ribs, tongue	1 oz.
Cheeses with 4–7 grams of fat per ounce: feta, mozzarella, pasteurized processed cheese spread, reduced-fat cheeses	1 oz.
Cheese, ricotta (regular or part-skim)	¼ cup (2 oz.)
Egg	1 egg
Fish: any fried	1 oz.
Lamb: ground, rib roast	1 oz.
Pork: cutlet, ground, shoulder roast	1 oz.
Poultry with skin: chicken, dove, pheasant, turkey, wild duck, or goose; fried chicken	1 oz.
Sausage with 4–7 grams of fat per ounce*	1 oz.

*High in sodium (based on the sodium content of a typical 3-ounce serving of meat, unless 1 ounce or 2 ounces is the normal serving size)

High-fat protein

These foods are high in saturated fat, cholesterol, and calories and may raise blood cholesterol levels if eaten on a regular basis. Try to eat three or fewer choices from this group per week.

One high-fat protein choice has 0 grams of carbohydrate, 7 grams of protein, 8 grams of fat, and 100 calories.

Note: The serving size for meat, fish, poultry, or hard cheeses is usually 1 ounce.

High-Fat Protein

Food	Serving Size
Bacon, pork	2 slices (1 oz. each before cooking)
Bacon, turkey*	3 slices (½ oz. each before cooking)
Cheese, regular: American, blue-veined, brie, cheddar, hard goat, Monterey jack, Parmesan, queso, Swiss	1 oz.

(continued)

(continued)

Food	Serving Size
Hot dog: beef, pork, or combination**	1 hot dog (10 hot dogs per 1-lb. package)
Hot dog: turkey or chicken	1 hot dog (10 hot dogs per 1-lb. package)
Pork: sausage, spareribs	1 oz.
Processed sandwich meats with 8 grams of fat or more per ounce: bologna, hard salami, pastrami*	1 oz.
Sausage with 8 grams fat or more per ounce: bratwurst, chorizo, Italian, knockwurst, Polish, smoked, summer*	1 oz.

High in sodium (based on the sodium content of a typical 3-ounce serving of meat, unless 1 ounce or 2 ounces is the normal serving size)
**Extra fat*

Plant-Based Protein

Food	Serving Size	Choices per Serving
"Bacon" strips, soy-based	2 strips (½ oz.)	1 lean protein
Baked beans, canned*	⅓ cup	1 starch + 1 lean protein
Beans (black, garbanzo, kidney, lima, navy, pinto, white), cooked or canned, drained and rinsed*	½ cup	1 starch + 1 lean protein
"Beef" or "sausage" crumbles, meatless	1 oz.	1 lean protein
"Chicken" nuggets, soy-based	2 nuggets (1½ oz.)	½ carbohydrate + 1 medium-fat protein
Edamame, shelled*	½ cup	½ carbohydrate + 1 lean protein
Falafel (spiced chickpea and wheat patties)	3 patties (about 2 inches across)	1 carbohydrate + 1 high-fat protein
Hot dog, meatless, soy-based	1 hot dog (1½ oz.)	1 lean protein
Hummus*	⅓ cup	1 carbohydrate + 1 medium-fat protein
Lentils, any color, cooked or canned, drained and rinsed*	½ cup	1 starch + 1 lean protein
Meatless burger, soy-based	3 oz.	½ carbohydrate + 2 lean proteins

Food	Serving Size	Choices per Serving
Meatless burger, vegetable- and starch-based*	1 patty (about 2½ oz.)	½ carbohydrate + 1 lean protein
Meatless deli slices	1 oz.	1 lean protein
Mycoprotein ("chicken" tenders or crumbles), meatless	2 oz.	½ carbohydrate + 1 lean protein
Nut spreads: almond butter, cashew butter, peanut butter, soy nut butter	1 tablespoon	1 high-fat protein
Peas (black-eyed and split peas), cooked or canned, drained and rinsed*	½ cup	1 starch + 1 lean protein
Refried beans, canned*/**	½ cup	1 starch + 1 lean protein
"Sausage" breakfast-type patties, meatless	1 (1½ oz.)	1 medium-fat protein
Soy nuts, unsalted	¾ oz.	½ carbohydrate + 1 medium-fat protein
Tempeh, plain, unflavored	¼ cup (1½ oz.)	1 medium-fat protein
Tofu	½ cup (4 oz.)	1 medium-fat protein
Tofu, light	½ cup (4 oz.)	1 lean protein

Note: *Because carbohydrate content varies among plant-based protein foods, read food labels.*
*Good source of fiber
**High in sodium (based on the sodium content of a typical 3-ounce serving of meat, unless 1 ounce or 2 ounces is the normal serving size)

Fats

One fat choice has 5 grams of fat and 45 calories.

Unsaturated Fats: Monounsaturated

Food	Serving Size
Almond milk (unsweetened)	1 cup
Avocado, medium	2 tablespoons (1 oz.)
Nut butters (trans fat–free): almond butter, cashew butter, peanut butter (smooth or crunchy)	1½ teaspoons
Nuts, almonds	6 nuts

(continued)

(continued)

Food	Serving Size
Nuts, Brazil	2 nuts
Nuts, cashews	6 nuts
Nuts, filberts (hazelnuts)	5 nuts
Nuts, macadamia	3 nuts
Nuts, mixed (50% peanuts)	6 nuts
Nuts, peanuts	10 nuts
Nuts, pecans	4 halves
Nuts, pistachios	16 nuts
Oil: canola, olive, peanut	1 teaspoon
Olives, black (ripe)	8
Olives, green, stuffed	10 large
Spread, plant stanol ester–type, light	1 tablespoon
Spread, plant stanol ester–type, regular	2 teaspoons

Unsaturated Fats: Polyunsaturated

Food	Serving Size
Margarine, lower-fat spread (30%–50% vegetable oil, trans fat–free)	1 tablespoon
Margarine, stick, tub (trans fat–free), or squeeze (trans fat–free)	1 teaspoon
Mayonnaise, reduced-fat	1 tablespoon
Mayonnaise, regular	1 teaspoon
Mayonnaise-style salad dressing, reduced-fat	1 tablespoon
Mayonnaise-style salad dressing, regular	2 teaspoon
Nuts, pignolia (pine nuts)	1 tablespoon
Nuts, walnuts, English	4 halves
Oil: corn, cottonseed, flaxseed, grapeseed, safflower, soybean, sunflower	1 teaspoon
Salad dressing, reduced-fat*	2 tablespoons
Salad dressing, regular	1 tablespoon

Food	Serving Size
Seeds, flaxseed, ground	1½ tablespoons
Seeds, pumpkin, sesame, sunflower	1 tablespoon
Tahini or sesame paste	2 teaspoons

May contain carbohydrate.

Saturated Fats

Food	Serving Size
Bacon, cooked, regular or turkey	1 slice
Butter, reduced-fat	1 tablespoon
Butter, stick	1 teaspoon
Butter, whipped	2 teaspoons
Butter blends made with oil, reduced-fat or light	1 tablespoon
Butter blends made with oil, regular	1½ teaspoons
Chitterlings, boiled	2 tablespoons (½ oz.)
Coconut, sweetened, shredded	2 tablespoons
Coconut milk, canned, thick, light	⅓ cup
Coconut milk, canned, thick, regular	1½ tablespoons
Coconut milk beverage (thin), unsweetened	1 cup
Cream, half-and-half	2 tablespoons
Cream, heavy	1 tablespoon
Cream, light	1½ tablespoons
Cream, whipped	2 tablespoons
Cream cheese, reduced-fat	1½ tablespoons (¾ oz.)
Cream cheese, regular	1 tablespoon (½ oz.)
Lard	1 teaspoon
Oil: coconut, palm, palm kernel	1 teaspoon
Salt pork	¼ oz.
Shortening, solid	1 teaspoon
Sour cream, reduced-fat or light	3 tablespoons
Sour cream, regular	2 tablespoons

Free Foods

If a "free" food is listed with a serving size, that means the calories and/or carbohydrate are near the limits defined for "free." Limit yourself to 3 servings or fewer
of that food per day, and spread the servings throughout the day. If you eat all
3 servings at once, the carbohydrate in the food may raise your blood glucose level
like 1 carbohydrate choice would. Food and drink choices listed here without a
serving size can be used whenever you like.

Low-Carbohydrate Foods

Food	Serving Size
Candy, hard (regular or sugar-free)	1 piece
Fruits, cranberries or rhubarb, sweetened with sugar substitute	½ cup
Gelatin dessert, sugar-free, any flavor	
Gum, sugar-free	
Jam or jelly, light or no-sugar-added	2 teaspoons
Salad greens (such as arugula, chicory, endive, escarole, leaf or iceberg lettuce, purslane, romaine, radicchio, spinach, watercress)	
Sugar substitutes (artificial sweeteners)	
Syrup, sugar-free	2 tablespoons
Vegetables: any raw nonstarchy vegetables (such as broccoli, cabbage, carrots, cucumber, tomato)	½ cup
Vegetables: any cooked nonstarchy vegetables (such as carrots, cauliflower, green beans)	¼ cup

Reduced-Fat or Fat-Free Foods

Food	Serving Size
Cream cheese, fat-free	1 tablespoon (½ oz.)
Coffee creamers, nondairy, liquid, flavored	1½ teaspoons
Coffee creamers, nondairy, liquid, sugar-free, flavored	4 teaspoons
Coffee creamers, nondairy, powdered, flavored	1 teaspoon
Coffee creamers, nondairy, powdered, sugar-free, flavored	2 teaspoons
Margarine spread, fat-free	1 tablespoon
Margarine spread, reduced-fat	1 teaspoon

Food	Serving Size
Mayonnaise, fat-free	1 tablespoon
Mayonnaise, reduced-fat	1 teaspoon
Mayonnaise-style salad dressing, fat-free	1 tablespoon
Mayonnaise-style salad dressing, reduced-fat	2 teaspoons
Salad dressing, fat-free	1 tablespoon
Salad dressing, fat-free, Italian	2 tablespoons
Sour cream, fat-free or reduced-fat	1 tablespoon
Whipped topping, light or fat-free	2 tablespoons
Whipped topping, regular	1 tablespoon

Condiments

Food	Serving Size
Barbecue sauce	2 teaspoons
Catsup (ketchup)	1 tablespoon
Chili sauce, sweet, tomato-type	2 teaspoons
Horseradish	
Hot pepper sauce	
Lemon juice	
Miso	1½ teaspoons
Mustard, honey	1 tablespoon
Mustard, brown, Dijon, horseradish-flavored, wasabi-flavored, or yellow	
Parmesan cheese, grated	1 tablespoon
Pickle relish (dill or sweet)	1 tablespoon
Pickles, dill*	1½ medium pickles
Pickles, sweet, bread and butter	2 slices
Pickles, sweet, gherkin	¾ oz.
Pimento	
Salsa	¼ cup

(continued)

(continued)

Food	Serving Size
Soy sauce, light or regular*	1 tablespoon
Sweet-and-sour sauce	2 teaspoons
Taco sauce	1 tablespoon
Vinegar	
Worcestershire sauce	
Yogurt, any type	2 tablespoons

High in sodium

Drinks/Mixes

Bouillon, broth, consommé*

Bouillon or broth, low-sodium

Club soda

Cocoa powder, unsweetened (1 tablespoon)

Coffee, unsweetened or with sugar substitute

Diet soft drinks, sugar-free

Drink mixes (powder or liquid drops), sugar-free

Tea, unsweetened or with sugar substitute

Tonic water, sugar-free

Water

Water, flavored, sugar-free

Good source of fiber

Seasonings

Flavoring extracts (for example, vanilla, almond, or peppermint)

Garlic, fresh or powder

Herbs, fresh or dried

Kelp

Nonstick cooking spray

Spices

Wine, used in cooking

Combination Foods

Entrées

Food	Serving Size	Choices per Serving
Casserole-type entrees (tuna noodle, lasagna, spaghetti with meatballs, chili with beans, macaroni and cheese)*	1 cup (8 oz.)	2 carbohydrates + 2 medium-fat proteins
Stews (beef/other meats and vegetables)*	1 cup (8 oz.)	1 carbohydrate + 1 medium-fat protein + 0–3 fats

*High in sodium

Frozen Meals/Entrées

Food	Serving Size	Choices per Serving
Burrito (beef and bean)*/**	1 burrito (5 oz.)	3 carbohydrates + 1 lean protein + 2 fats
Dinner-type healthy meal (includes dessert and is usually less than 400 calories)	about 9–12 oz.	2–3 carbohydrates + 1–2 lean proteins + 1 fat
"Healthy"-type entree (usually less than 300 calories)	about 7–10 oz.	2 carbohydrates + 2 lean proteins
Pizza, cheese/vegetarian, thin crust**	¼ of a 12-inch pizza (4½–5 oz.)	2 carbohydrates + 2 medium-fat proteins
Pizza, meat topping, thin crust**	¼ of a 12-inch pizza (5 oz.)	2 carbohydrates + 2 medium-fat proteins + 1½ fats
Pizza, cheese/vegetarian or meat topping, rising crust**	⅙ of 12-inch pizza (4 oz.)	2½ carbohydrates + 2 medium-fat proteins
Pocket sandwich**	1 sandwich (4½ oz.)	3 carbohydrates + 1 lean protein + 1–2 fats
Pot pie**	1 pot pie (7 oz.)	3 carbohydrates + 1 medium-fat protein + 3 fats

*Good source of fiber
**High in sodium

Salads (Deli-Style)

Food	Serving Size	Choices per Serving
Coleslaw	½ cup	1 carbohydrate + 1½ fats
Macaroni/pasta salad	½ cup	2 carbohydrates + 3 fats
Potato salad*	½ cup	1½–2 carbohydrates + 1–2 fats
Tuna salad or chicken salad	½ cup (3½ oz.)	½ carbohydrate +2 lean proteins + 1 fat

*High in sodium

Soups

Food	Serving Size	Choices per Serving
Bean, lentil, or split pea soup*/**	1 cup (8 oz.)	1½ carbohydrates + 1 lean protein
Chowder (made with milk)**	1 cup (8 oz.)	1 carbohydrate + 1 lean protein + 1½ fats
Cream soup (made with water)**	1 cup (8 oz.)	1 carbohydrate + 1 fat
Miso soup**	1 cup (8 oz.)	½ carbohydrate + 1 lean protein
Ramen noodle soup**	1 cup (8 oz.)	2 carbohydrates + 2 fats
Rice soup/porridge (congee)	1 cup (8 oz.)	1 carbohydrate
Tomato soup (made with water), borscht**	1 cup (8 oz.)	1 carbohydrate
Vegetable beef, chicken noodle, or other broth-type soup (including "healthy"-type soups, such as those lower in sodium and/or fat)**	1 cup (8 oz.)	1 carbohydrate + 1 lean protein

*Good source of fiber

**High in sodium

Fast Foods

Main Dishes/Entrées

Food	Serving Size	Choices per Serving
Chicken, breast, breaded and fried*/****	1 (about 7 oz.)	1 carbohydrate + 6 medium-fat proteins
Chicken, breast, meat only**	1	4 lean proteins

Food	Serving Size	Choices per Serving
Chicken, drumstick, breaded and fried*	1 (about 2½ oz.)	½ carbohydrate + 2 medium-fat proteins
Chicken, drumstick, meat only**	1	1 lean protein + ½ fat
Chicken, nuggets or tenders****	6 (about 3½ oz.)	1 carbohydrate + 2 medium-fat proteins + 1 fat
Chicken, thigh, breaded and fried*/****	1 (about 5 oz.)	1 carbohydrate + 3 medium-fat proteins + 2 fats
Chicken, thigh, meat only**	1	2 lean proteins + ½ fat
Chicken, wing, breaded and fried*	1 wing (about 2 oz.)	½ carbohydrate + 2 medium-fat proteins
Chicken, wing, meat only**	1 wing	1 lean protein
Main dish salad (grilled chicken-type, no dressing or croutons)***/****	1 salad (about 11½ oz.)	1 carbohydrate + 4 lean proteins
Pizza, cheese, pepperoni, or sausage, regular or thick crust****	⅛ of a 14-inch pizza (about 4 oz.)	2½ carbohydrates + 1 high-fat protein + 1 fat
Pizza, cheese, pepperoni, or sausage, thin crust****	⅛ of a 14-inch pizza (about 2¾ oz.)	1½ carbohydrates + 1 high-fat protein + 1 fats
Pizza, cheese, meat, and vegetable, regular crust****	⅛ of a 14-inch pizza (about 5 oz.)	2½ carbohydrates + 2 high-fat proteins

*Definition and weight refer to food with bone, skin, and breading.
**Definition refers to food without bone, skin, and breading.
***Good source of fiber
****High in sodium

Asian

Food	Serving Size	Choices per Serving
Beef/chicken/shrimp with vegetables in sauce*	1 cup (about 6 oz.)	1 carbohydrate + 2 lean proteins + 1 fat
Egg roll, meat	1 egg roll (about 3 oz.)	1½ carbohydrates + 1 lean protein + 1½ fats
Fried rice, meatless	1 cup	2½ carbohydrates + 2 fats
Fortune cookie	1 cookie	½ carbohydrate
Hot-and-sour soup*	1 cup	½ carbohydrate + ½ fat

(continued)

(continued)

Food	Serving Size	Choices per Serving
Meat with sweet sauce*	1 cup (about 6 oz.)	3½ carbohydrates + 3 medium-fat proteins + 3 fats
Noodles and vegetables in sauce (chow mein, lo mein)*	1 cup	2 carbohydrates + 2 fats

High in sodium

Mexican

Food	Serving Size	Choices per Serving
Burrito with beans and cheese*/**	1 small burrito (about 6 oz.)	3½ carbohydrates + 1 medium-fat protein + 1 fat
Nachos with cheese**	1 small order (about 8 nachos)	2½ carbohydrates + 1 high-fat protein + 2 fats
Quesadilla, cheese only**	1 small order (about 5 oz.)	2½ carbohydrates + 3 high-fat proteins
Taco, crisp, with meat and cheese	1 small taco (about 3 oz.)	1 carbohydrate + 1 medium-fat protein + ½ fat
Taco salad with chicken and tortilla bowl*/**	1 salad (1 lb., including tortilla bowl)	3½ carbohydrates + 4 medium-fat proteins + 3 fats
Tostada with beans and cheese**	1 small tostada (about 5 oz.)	2 carbohydrates + 1 high-fat protein

Good source of fiber
**High in sodium*

Sandwiches

Food	Serving Size	Choices per Serving
Breakfast sandwich, breakfast burrito with sausage, egg, cheese*	1 burrito (about 4 oz.)	1½ carbohydrates + 2 high-fat proteins
Breakfast sandwich, egg, cheese, meat on an English muffin*	1 sandwich	2 carbohydrates + 3 medium-fat proteins + ½ fat
Breakfast sandwich, egg, cheese, meat on a biscuit*	1 sandwich	2 carbohydrates + 3 medium-fat proteins + 2 fats
Breakfast sandwich, sausage biscuit sandwich*	1 sandwich	2 carbohydrates + 1 high-fat protein + 4 fats
Chicken sandwich, grilled with bun, lettuce, tomatoes, spread*	1 sandwich (about 7½ oz.)	3 carbohydrates + 4 lean proteins

Food	Serving Size	Choices per Serving
Chicken sandwich, crispy, with bun, lettuce, tomatoes, spread*	1 sandwich (about 6 oz.)	3 carbohydrates + 2 lean proteins + 3½ fats
Chicken sandwich, fish sandwich with tartar sauce and cheese	1 sandwich (5 oz.)	2½ carbohydrates + 2 medium-fat proteins + 1½ fats
Hamburger, regular with bun and condiments (ketchup, mustard, onion, pickle)	1 burger (about 3½ oz.)	2 carbohydrates + 1 medium-fat protein + 1 fat
Hamburger, 4 oz. meat with cheese, bun, and condiments (ketchup, mustard, onion, pickle)*	1 burger (about 8½ oz.)	3 carbohydrates + 4 medium-fat protein + 2½ fats
Hot dog with bun, plain*	1 hot dog (about 3½ oz.)	1½ carbohydrates + 1 high-fat protein + 2 fats
Submarine sandwich (no cheese or sauce), less than 6 grams fat*	One 6-inch sub	3 carbohydrates + 2 lean proteins
Submarine sandwich (no cheese or sauce), regular*	One 6-inch sub	3 carbohydrates + 2 lean proteins + 1 fat
Wrap, grilled chicken, vegetables, cheese, and spread*	1 small wrap (about 4–5 oz.)	2 carbohydrates + 2 lean proteins + 1½ fats

*High in sodium

Sides/Appetizers

Food	Serving Size	Choices per Serving
French fries*/**	1 small order (about 3½ oz.)	2½ carbohydrates + 2 fats
French fries*/**	1 medium order (about 5 oz.)	3½ carbohydrates + 3 fats
French fries*/**	1 large order (about 6 oz.)	4½ carbohydrates + 4 fats
Hashbrowns**	1 cup/medium order (about 5 oz.)	3 carbohydrates + 6 fats
Onion rings**	1 serving (8–9 rings, about 4 oz.)	3½ carbohydrates + 4 fats
Salad, side (no dressing, croutons or cheese)	1 small salad	1 nonstarchy vegetable

*Extra fat
**High in sodium

Beverages and Desserts

Food	Serving Size	Choices per Serving
Coffee, latte (fat-free milk)	1 small order (about 12 oz.)	1 fat-free milk
Coffee, mocha (fat-free milk, no whipped cream)	1 small order (about 12 oz.)	1 fat-free milk + 1 carbohydrate
Milkshake, any flavor	1 small shake (about 12 oz.)	5½ carbohydrates + 3 fats
Milkshake, any flavor	1 medium shake (about 16 oz.)	7 carbohydrates + 4 fats
Milkshake, any flavor	1 large shake (about 22 oz.)	10 carbohydrates + 5 fats
Soft-serve ice cream cone	1 small	2 carbohydrates + ½ fat

Alcohol

One alcohol equivalent or choice (½ oz. absolute alcohol) has about 100 calories. One carbohydrate choice has 15 grams of carbohydrate and about 70 calories.

Alcoholic Beverage	Serving Size	Choices per Serving
Beer, light (less than 4.5% abv)	12 fl. oz.	1 alcohol equivalent + ½ carbohydrate
Beer, regular (about 5% abv)	12 fl. oz.	1 alcohol equivalent + 1 carbohydrate
Beer, dark (more than 5.7% abv)	12 fl. oz.	1 alcohol equivalent + 1–1½ carbohydrates
Distilled spirits (80 or 86 proof): vodka, rum, gin, whiskey, tequila	1½ fl. oz.	1 alcohol equivalent
Liqueur, coffee (53 proof)	1 fl. oz.	½ alcohol equivalent + 1 carbohydrate
Sake	1 fl. oz.	½ alcohol equivalent
Wine, champagne/sparkling	5 fl. oz.	1 alcohol equivalent
Wine, dessert (sherry)	3½ fl. oz.	1 alcohol equivalent + 1 carbohydrate
Wine, dry, red or white (10% abv)	5 fl. oz.	1 alcohol equivalent

Note: *% abv refers to the percentage of alcohol by volume.*

Index

Couscous Salad recipe, 159

Crab and Rice Salad recipe, 160

Crab Imperial recipe, 126

Crab-Filled Mushrooms recipe, 145

crackers, on Starch food list, 309–310

Cream of Carrot Soup recipe, 57

Creamy Cheese Dip recipe, 152

Creamy Herb Dressing recipe, 174

Creole Steak recipe, 105

Crêpes Suzette recipe, 228

Crumb Pie Shell recipe, 229

Cucumber Pâté recipe, 146

Curried Rice with Pineapple recipe, 200

D

dairy, 18

DASH (Dietary Approaches to Stop Hypertension) eating plan, 279, 281

deli meat, 32

deprivation, 295

desserts
  about, 217
  on Fast Foods food list, 334
  recipes for, 218–241

diabetes food choices/exchanges method, of meal planning
  about, 250, 269
  food lists, 270–276
  using, 276–277
  what they are, 270

diabetes-friendly eating patterns method, of meal planning, 250

"diabetic" food, 31

Dietary Approaches to Stop Hypertension (DASH) eating plan, 279, 281

dietary fiber, 267

dietitians
  certified diabetes educators (CDEs), 248, 280
  meeting with, 248–249
  registered dietitian (RD), 29, 248, 280
  registered dietitian nutritionist (RDN), 29, 248, 280
  talking to, 290

Dill Dressing recipe, 175

dining out. See eating out

doughnuts, on Sweets, Desserts, and Other Carbohydrates food list, 318

dressings. See salads and dressings

dried fruit, 11

dried herbs, 24

dried spices, 24

drinks
  about, 18–20
  alcohol, 19–20, 334
  on Fast Foods food list, 334
  on Free Foods food list, 328
  on Sweets, Desserts, and Other Carbohydrates food list, 315–316

dry food, 26–27

E

eating healthy. See healthy eating

eating out
  about, 297
  asking your server, 298
  creativity when, 301–302
  drinks, 301
  extras, 300
  fast food, 302–303
  researching restaurants, 298
  special requests, 299
  substitutions and, 299–300
  take-home containers, 301
  takeout, 302

eating patterns
  Dietary Approaches to Stop Hypertension (DASH) eating plan, 279, 281
  low-carbohydrate eating patterns, 279, 283
  low-fat eating patterns, 279, 284
  meal planning and, 280–284
  Mediterranean-style eating plan, 279, 280–281
  plant-based (vegetarian/vegan) eating patterns, 279, 282–283

Eggplant Lasagna recipe, 71

eggs, 34

English Beef Stew recipe, 58

entrées
- on Combination Foods food list, 329
- on Fast Foods food list, 330–331

Environmental Protection Agency, 13

essentials, stocking up on, 23–28

events, snacking before, 294

expectations, managing, 39

F

fast food, 302–303

Fast Foods food list, 276, 330–334

fat-free foods, on Free Foods food list, 326–327

fat(s)
- about, 15
- in alcohol, 306
- in Fats food list choices, 275, 306
- in Fruit food list choices, 271, 305
- healthy, 17–18, 247–248
- importance of, 247–248
- in Milk and Milk Substitutes food list choices, 272, 305
- in Nonstarchy Vegetables food list choices, 273, 306
- in Protein food list choices, 274, 306
- reducing, 36
- saturated, 266, 275, 325
- in Starch food list choices, 271, 305
- in Sweets, Desserts, and Other Carbohydrates food list choices, 273, 306
- trans, 16, 266, 275
- unhealthy, 15–16
- unsaturated, 275, 323–325

Fats food list, 274–275, 323–325

Festive Sweet Potatoes recipe, 201

Fettuccine with Peppers and Broccoli recipe, 72

fiber, dietary, 267

Fiery Black Bean Salad recipe, 157

fish, 13

flavor, 36–37

Flounder Parmesan recipe, 127

Food and Drug Administration, 13

food lists
- about, 270, 305–306
- Combination Foods, 275–276, 329–330
- Fast Foods, 276, 330–334
- Fats, 274–275, 323–325
- Free Foods, 275, 326–328
- Fruits, 271–272, 310–313
- Milk and Milk Substitutes, 272, 313–314
- Nonstarchy vegetables, 272–273, 314–315
- Protein, 274, 319–323
- Starch, 270–271, 306–310
- Sweets, Desserts, and Other Carbohydrates, 273, 315–319

food(s)
- canned, 26–27
- carbohydrates, 8, 247
- dairy, 18
- drinks, 18–20
- dry, 26–27
- fat, 15–18
- fresh, 27–28
- fruit, 10–11
- grains, 11–12, 26
- protein, 12–15
- vegetables, 8, 181
- what to eat, 7–20

Free Foods food list, 275, 326–328

French Dressing recipe, 176

Fresh Apple Pie recipe, 230

Fresh Blueberry Pancakes recipe, 45

Fresh Dill Dip recipe, 147

Fresh Fish Chowder recipe, 59

fresh food, 27–28

frozen bars, on Sweets, Desserts, and Other Carbohydrates food list, 318–319

frozen desserts, on Sweets, Desserts, and Other Carbohydrates food list, 318–319

frozen meals/entrées, on Combination Foods food list, 329

frozen yogurt, on Sweets, Desserts, and Other Carbohydrates food list, 318–319

Lamb Chops with Orange Sauce recipe, 109

lean protein, on Protein food list, 319–320

Lemon Chicken recipe, 89

Lentil Salad recipe, 164

Lentil Soup recipe, 61

lentils, on Starch food list, 310

Light Hollandaise recipe, 178

Linguine with Pesto Sauce recipe, 77

Lobster Fricassee recipe, 132

Lobster Salad recipe, 165

Low-Calorie, Fat-Free Whipped Cream recipe, 232

low-carbohydrate eating patterns, 279, 283

low-carbohydrate foods, on Free Foods food list, 326

Low-Fat Cream Cheese Frosting recipe, 233

low-fat eating patterns, 279, 284

M

macronutrients
  about, 246
  carbohydrates as, 247
  fat as, 247–248
  protein as, 247

main dishes/entrées, on Fast Foods food list, 330–331

Make-Ahead Apple, Carrot, and Cabbage Slaw recipe, 167

Manhattan Clam Chowder recipe, 64

Marinara Sauce recipe, 80

Marinated Leg of Lamb recipe, 110

marinating protein, 36

Marvelous Meat Loaf recipe, 111

mayonnaise, 34

meal planning
  about, 245–246, 279
  dietitians, 248–249
  eating patterns and, 280–284
  macronutrients, 246–248
  variety in, 249–250

meat
  deli, 32
  red, 14–15
  substitutes for, 14, 283

Mediterranean Chicken Salad recipe, 166

Mediterranean -Style Chicken Scaloppine recipe, 82

Mediterranean-style eating plan, 279, 280–281

Mediterranean-Style Scalloped Potatoes recipe, 205

medium-fat protein, on Protein food list, 320–321

Mexican food, on Fast Foods food list, 332

Mexican Tortilla Soup recipe, 62

microwaving, 35

milk
  about, 34
  on Milk and Milk Substitutes food list, 313

Milk and Milk Substitutes food list, 272, 313–314

milk foods, on Milk and Milk Substitutes food list, 314

milk substitutes, on Milk and Milk Substitutes food list, 314

mindless eating, 292

Mini Breakfast Quiches recipe, 49

mixes, on Free Foods food list, 328

monounsaturated fats, on Fats food list, 323–324

Monterey Jack Cheese Quiche Squares recipe, 153

muffins. *See* breads and muffins

Mushroom Cassoulets recipe, 189

N

neotame, 25

nonstarchy vegetables
  about, 9
  carbohydrates in, 260
  Plate Method and, 254–255

Nonstarchy Vegetables food list, 272–273, 314–315

Nutrition Facts label, 264–267, 291

"Nutrition Therapy Recommendations for the Management of Adults with Diabetes," 284

nuts, 275

O

Oatmeal Raisin Cookies recipe, 234

oils, 23

Oldways Whole Grain Council, 12

tortillas, 34

trans fats
about, 16, 275
on nutrition panels, 266

trans fatty acids, 16

Turkey Burgers recipe, 100

Turkey Sausage Patties recipe, 50

Turkey with Almond Duxelles recipe, 101

U

unhealthy fats, 15–16

unsaturated fats
about, 275
on Fats food list, 323–325

V

veal
about, 14, 103
recipes for, 104–117

Veal Romano recipe, 116

Veal Scaloppine recipe, 117

Vegetable Lo Mein recipe, 79

vegetables
about, 8, 181
aromatic, 37
nonstarchy, 9, 254–255, 260
on Nonstarchy Vegetables food list, 314–315
recipes for, 182–195
replacing protein with, 34
starchy, 9–10, 308–309

Vegetable-Stuffed Yellow Squash recipe, 194

vegetarian/vegan (plant-based) eating patterns, 282–283

W

Walnut Macaroons recipe, 241

Warning icon, 3

websites
Cheat Sheet, 4
Environmental Protection Agency, 13
Food and Drug Administration, 13
Whole Grain Stamp, 12

Western Omelet recipe, 51

White Bean Soup recipe, 68

Whole Grain Stamp (website), 12

Wild Rice Salad recipe, 171

Wine-Poached Chicken with Herbs and Vegetables recipe, 97

Y

yogurt
full-fat, 32
on Milk and Milk Substitutes food list, 313

Z

Zucchini, Carrot, and Fennel Salad recipe, 172

Zucchini Sauté recipe, 195

About the Author

The American Diabetes Association is the nation's leading nonprofit organization fighting diabetes and its consequences. The Association's mission is to prevent and cure diabetes and to improve the lives of all people affected by diabetes. We work toward this mission by funding research to prevent, cure, and manage all types of diabetes; providing services to people and communities affected by diabetes and reliable information to patients and healthcare providers; and advocating for the rights of people with diabetes. For more information, please visit www.diabetes.org or call 800-DIABETES (800-342-2383).

Acknowledgments

The American Diabetes Association would like to acknowledge Amy Riolo for preparing the incredible recipes in this book. Thank you for showing people with diabetes how unbelievably easy it can be to create delicious, healthy meals at home. We'd also like to thank Tracy Boggier, Senior Acquisitions Editor at Wiley, and Vicki Adang, of Mark My Words Editorial Services, LLC, for managing this project, as well as Elizabeth Kuball for her thorough editorial work. Your ideas, guidance, and support have been invaluable to this process.

Publisher's Acknowledgments

Senior Acquisitions Editor: Tracy Boggier

Project Editor: Elizabeth Kuball

Copy Editor: Elizabeth Kuball

Production Editor: Antony Sami

Cover Image: © Chris Christou/Shutterstock

Special Help: Victoria M. Adang